CONFESSIONS OF A FAST FOOD FREAK

(But I still lost 40 lbs in 90 days eating at McDonald's 90% of the time)

DD ANDER

www.ddander.com

Legal Notes

ISBN number: 978-0-9953193-2-5

AND SO IT BEGINS

I have had, and still have, an ongoing affair with McD's that has outlasted several significant relationships and shows no signs of abating anytime soon. I dine out on a regular basis and that is unlikely to change, at least in the foreseeable future. BUT THIS I KNOW: I NEED TO LOSE WEIGHT! NOW!

I'm on a runaway going the wrong way fast! But, I also know me, and I've decided that I might just as well admit to the following facts:

1. I'm going to eat at McD's and that is just the way it is!
2. I rarely, if ever, cook for myself. I eat out.
3. I'm not going to suddenly start eating salads and the like; it ain't gonna happen!
4. I am pretty sure I'm addicted to Diet Coke! Horrors!
5. I'm a meat eater and an egg eater, and McD's has plenty of these.

6. I consider myself to be reasonable intelligent, so yes, I've read the literature; every nasty article and study known to man!

7. McD's is my microcosm. I meet clients here; I meet friends, and friends yet unmade, in this place. I write here; I study here, and so on!

8. Did I mention it has WIFI?

9. I am alone a great deal of the time and this place is comforting to me. I know the staff well, and many of the regular clientele.

10. I have my favourite spot(s) where I can plug in my iPad and disappear into cyberspace for as long as I want.

11. I believe that this place is allowing me to pursue a higher purpose.

12. This is my SAFE place. I am not a transient, yet in my own mind, I am, for my home is very far away. I will go home one day. Just not yet.

13. Here are some US stats: 50,000,000 people are served daily in fast food restaurants. Of that number, 10,000,000 (20%) people eat fast food twice per week. 7,000,000 (14%) eat it 3 or more times weekly, and 3,000,000 (6%)

eat fast food 7 times per week. (reported in Oct. 2015 by www.statisticbrain.com)

14. We are not alone. The top 5 consumers of fast food are the United States, France, Canada, United Kingdom, and South Korea as reported by www.countryranker.com in Aug. 2015

Let me tell you a little more. I admit that I'm somewhat out of sorts. My wife, and our home, is over 6,000 miles (10,000 km) from where I find myself. This is where the work is, but the milk and honey have not flowed nearly fast enough to allow my exit to be with the woman I love. So we bide our time. Patience has not been my greatest virtue, but endure I must, and endure I will!

In the meantime, I try to keep myself occupied in "safe" endeavours and in my "safe house." Oh McD's, how I love you!

I don't smoke or do drugs. I'm at best, a very casual drinker, in fact, essentially a non drinker, except for copious amounts of Diet Coke (aspartame and all)!

In the past I could get away with eating whatever I wanted because I worked hard, and I played even harder! I loved the hard workouts, especially on the racquet courts, and running the trails for miles at a time. I felt invincible, but over time, my body began to break down. A broken ankle, a fractured fibula, a shoulder used and abused far too much, a hernia, and general abuse of this instrument known as my body, finally began to damper my desire to "play" hard. I accepted that fact less than graciously, but even though I was forced to "slow down", the one area that did not go along with the "new" me was the eating habits. And the evidence became hard to ignore!

I ate whatever I wanted, and lots of it! And it began to take its toll! Soon I was heavy, embarrassingly so, and it became a never ending story. I would rebound from time to time, but inevitably, I would regain all the weight I'd lost and add some more for good measure.

Do you relate? I know I am not alone in this ongoing battle with the dark side! I also know that today is the day that I will once again confront my demons! I don't feel like it; I don't want to; but I have to! I have to at least try! So I will put fingers to keypad and record my life on a daily basis. I need to make it a competition of sorts or I will fail once again before I even get started. I need the time frame to be long enough to get results but short enough to keep me interested.

I've decided to set up the competition into 40 Day segments. That may seem like a short time to some of you but to anyone struggling with any kind of an addiction, food or otherwise, even 1 day can seem incredibly long. Why 40 Days? Simple. If Christ could endure 40 days in the desert alone without food and water, and have to put up with none other than Satan himself, I should be able to manage 40 days in my rather easy life. We shall see.

THE FIRST TEN DAYS - STAGE 1

Day 1. I weigh 272 pounds! I've gained 40 pounds over the last 3 years, and if I don't get a handle on this runaway freight train, I see a 300 pound future, short though it may be!

I should have started my day with a long walk in the park but I didn't. Instead, I went to McD's and read the paper, did a little research on a project, and consumed 2 large Diet Coke and an Egg McMuffin in the process.

I'm not as busy as I should be. I'd like to believe that it's strictly "the economy," but I'm not sure that that is the case. I say I want to "go home" and yet my actions belie my words. So I hide, usually at McD's . . .

I've never let fear be my guide, although on many occasions I probably should have. Instead, I would forge ahead. As a result I experienced life on my own terms and grew to appreciate the incredible diversity that mankind offers up. I think I can safely say that prejudice is not part of my vocabulary. I've always believed that we are all the same, and the same blood courses through all our veins.

Even so, the last number of years has offered up its own version of reality and my confidence in my abilities has been sorely tested. Where I once thought I could do anything, I've found that the faith I once had in myself was rapidly being replaced by fear instead. Paralyzing fear. I found that I was talking the talk but not walking the walk. Did I not want this new life that I had crossed mountain peaks and oceans to find?

It's not that I disappeared into myself; it's just that I wasn't performing at the economic level I needed to if I was making an International move. There were people counting on me and I needed to step up big time!

I found myself alone a lot, not necessarily lonely, but becoming increasingly impatient with my progress.

I drove by the trails just a short while ago thinking that I just might go for a stroll. But no, I managed to talk myself out of that crazy idea. I am consistent, if nothing else!

But I wasn't done yet! Oh no! Back to McD's I went and instead of a walk, I settled for a McDouble, small fries, and Diet Coke and followed that up a couple of hours later with a peanut butter sandwich and a bag of cheezies. My state of mind is not good. Thus ends day 1!

Day 2. I may have gotten off too a bad start but at least I started. I will reluctantly invite you more and more into my world as time goes by. We all have our struggles. I know I certainly do. It's a long and winding road that I traverse. I have been on this road for several years now and I know it well. Even so, I dare not lose sight of the lantern held aloft by the maiden at the other end beckoning me to come home. So, I make my way but it is taking far longer than I expected and that saddens me and it saddens her. So I eat to ease the pain. Brilliant! There are times that I think I am so intelligent and then there are times when the bulb is rather dim.

It's noon. I'm at McD's at the moment but I haven't decided whether to have a bite or not. In the meantime I write and pour forth that which I am compelled to share.

I used to be in great shape a few years back. There was nothing I wouldn't tackle. Everything I did was designed to increase endurance. With endurance comes confidence, and I knew that regardless of what I faced, I would endure. I'm not so sure of that anymore, in fact, I'm quite confident that I wouldn't endure if push came to shove. And that sucks!

I have a thousand reasons to endure, to run the good race. There is much to do in this world gone wrong and I want to do my part. I'm doing what I can while I'm here but I feel strongly that Panama is calling my name. And for that, endurance is a necessity. So, I will leave yesterday in the past where it belongs and start anew again today.

It's 5 pm and I'm at McD's again. Writing, and yes, I had a Quarter Pounder with Cheese, small fries, and Diet Coke. Hopefully that's it for the evening. After all, Day 1 was a disaster! (Confession: I went home and finished off a bag of cheezies and a cheese sandwich)

Day 3. Back to McD's this am. I'm cutting back so all I had was a Sausage, Egg and Cheese McMuffin and a Diet Coke.

Well, I was doing pretty good until lunch time. But then I went for lunch at the church. I pigged out on 2 hamburgers, 2 slices of ham, a fried egg, cheese, salad, and cheese cake (I don't even eat cheese cake!). Oh boy!

Then I went for a walk, a 2 mile (3km) stroll. We have a beautiful park system here. In days past, I ran these trails regularly, logging at least 10 miles (16 km) daily and I loved it! I was in great shape and endurance had indeed become my middle name! That was yesterday, but I'm determined to make it my tomorrow as well!

Of course, it was time to eat again and a huge plate of Chinese food found its way to my stomach.

3 days have now passed and I have not done well. I hope I am brave enough to continue on this journey. I want to start over and pretend the last three days didn't happen but that would be a mistake. I need to see this through. I need to suck it up. And I will!

Day 4. I need to get it together! It's pretty obvious to me that mentally I'm shot at the moment. To be perfectly honest, I'm feeling pretty insecure right now. For a guy that supposedly "has it all" according to some well meaning friends, I'm close to walking away from it all!

I'm getting more discouraged with each passing day. I'm starting to withdraw. I'm trying to hold on for dear life but I'm not sure how well I'm doing. Lord, I need you big time! I'm not particularly fond of me right now. Help me to quit this negative self talk, please! I may clean up well and present this wonderful image to those around me, but it's nothing more than a farce! I think I need help.

I've been to McD's twice today already. Let's see: Egg McMufffin, bran muffin, McDouble, small fries, several Diet Coke, and the day is not over.

Weight is something I've struggled with throughout the years. Most of the people I know never considered it to be much of a problem. You see, I carry my weight pretty well so only I know about the "hidden" 30 pounds or so that no one sees. But, I know that it's there, and I know its' effects. And I must admit, vanity does play a rather large role!

So, I've been up and I've been down, and when I'm on, I'm really on and in great shape. In the past, I would jog or play racquetball with a vengeance. I would strive constantly to "endure", to win, to outlast the competition even if I was my own competitor!

A particular trying time in my life found me at an all time high (or should I say low) of 305 pounds (138.6 kg)! Unbelievable, but oh so true! I fought back and I fought hard, and through sheer will power, I slowly regained my life. In fact, I went down too low, dropping to around 190 pounds (86.4 kg). I looked great and I felt great but I was weak and that would never do. I regained a few controlled pounds and settled in at about 205 pounds (93.2 kg) which turned out to be perfect for me. I was strong; I was fast; I was alive, and I was determined to never gain the weight back again! But, I was wrong. So wrong!

All it took was an injury or two along the way and I'd be taken down for a time. But in that downtime, I'd eat, and I'd eat a lot! I began to regain those pounds of yesterday quickly. When I was in great fighting shape I could eat anything and everything because I knew I could work it off. Now I was eating lots and exercising little, and the results were beginning to show. 10 pounds (4.5 kg) here, 10 pounds (4.5 kg) there, and soon I was up 50 pounds (22.7 kg). The pounds I had lost had found their way home. There are probably many of you reading my tale of woe who know exactly of what I speak!

And of course, I no longer felt like working out, or going for a run. It was a lot easier to make a sandwich and watch TV in my man cave. Besides, I was embarrassed about how I looked!

Over the years the cycle would repeat; up, down, up, down, ad nauseam. Today I find myself weighing in at 272 pounds (123.6 kg) and I am disgusted with myself!

Day 4 is coming to a close and once again I'm at McD's drinking a large Diet Coke. My stomach is upset although I'm not sure why. It's not like I upset it by eating anything really healthy, that's for sure!

THREE AND ONE HALF YEARS AGO

Three and one half years ago I decided to make a major change in my life. It was time for me to go. I was fed up with our way of life, with the blatant materialism, with the constant comparison of stuff which seemed to define us as successful or not. So I left! A one way ticket into Mexico and points beyond would be my salvation or at least point me away from a world gone mad. Or at least that's how I saw it. Even so, I took 250 pounds (113.6 kg) with me, as well as a wad of cash. I couldn't say for sure if this was a one way trip or not and I didn't really care! I just wanted to go, and I did!

I decided that I would go wherever I felt like on this so called Journey of Discovery and I'd do whatever I pleased. I soon found myself in Cozumel in scuba gear expecting to join the Cousteau's in the elusive search for Atlantis! But, something was off, and try as I might, I could not maintain equilibrium. It made no sense. I had swam a lot in my youth, in fact, I was a strong swimmer but now I was having a hard time staying down regardless of how much I adjusted the air pressure or piled on the weights. In any case, I decided to move on. I encountered the same issue in Belize and Panama whenever I would attempt to head to the bottom of the sea. It was only later that it all began to make sense.

Day 5. Sunday. Despite myself, I'm beginning to get some good results. I will post these at the end of each 10 day period, regardless of how good, bad, or ugly they are. I know that the biggest obstacle that I need to overcome is me. I know I'm not in a great space. Interestingly enough, I just came from a great service appropriately titled: Unstoppable Life . . . stress relief for today, tomorrow, and beyond. I already know this stuff but more action is required!

So it's off to McD's once again. I had my usual Egg McMuffin as well as a breakfast burrito and my customary Diet Coke. We will see where this leads to today.

I think it's time for a walk. I sure wish someone would give me a call. I wonder about my friends sometimes. Most of them know I spend a lot of time alone, and most of them know that I am struggling with loneliness at this time and yet, here I am.

Alone again. I know that I can pick up the phone and call them, and I often do, but so can they. I'm not one to have a pity party but I must confess, I'm kind of there right now.

Oh well. I'll put on my happy face and go about my business. How many times have I heard "you are always so happy! It's such a pleasure being around you!" Uh huh. Ok, I'll quit whining now!

Day 6. Mentally and emotionally I'm shot. But, a hot shower and a trip to my watering hole and I'm starting to feel a whole lot better. A friend just called and needs some assistance. Why not? That takes the focus off me, a least for a little while.

I had my McMuffin and hash brown earlier today and soon followed that up with a McDouble, small fries and Diet Coke. Of course, I had to have a soft ice cream cone as well.

I decided to go for another walk through our beautiful park. An hour and a half later I reluctantly called it a day. I felt great and I'd managed to capture a few wonderful photos. Now, if I can just keep this up! I may be down and somewhat discouraged but I haven't given up, and I won't!

I headed over to the church for CR (celebrate recovery), a program celebrating those who meet their hurts, hang ups, and habits head on, for some fellowship and teaching. Good stuff and definitely a lifeline in this troubling time. Of course, dinner was being served and I wasn't about to pass that up!

I am sore. I used to run these trails on a daily basis and certainly a lot farther than this little jaunt today. I mourn little for the past but I sure miss the old physical me. I find that depressing and that's when I'm closest to the abyss. When I stared down from the bridge today into the water below, the memories came rushing back, and I remember promising myself that I would never get out of shape again! Nothing stopped me. Weather be damned! In fact, I loved running in the rain. I owned the park on those runs, save for the odd runner or dog walker who loved the rain as much as I did.

But so what? At least I did it. I may not be in the condition of yesterday but I'm trying. I'm trying hard, and the memories stirred up will hopefully help propel me forward.

Day 7. I am not doing well. Even a hot bath and lots of prayer is failing to calm me down. From all appearances I look fine and totally in control. Beneath the surface I feel close to boiling over. I won't. Not me . . . Maybe.

I think I'd better make a call today.I'm almost robotic at the moment. I await . . . for what? The call that's going to change my life? Even I have a hard time believing that right now. And yet, it could be true. I know God has a plan for my life, and it certainly isn't to live my life the way I am right now! Lord, reveal yourself to me. I desperately need you right now!

So it's off to McD's once again. My "safe" place, perhaps too safe. Perhaps I need to "coffee" elsewhere, you know, shake it up a little. Sorry, that ain't going to happen.

I absolutely, positively need to stab this real estate career through the heart once and for all. It promises me big things but rarely delivers. It's a seductress and I am in its' power. It's got great potential; I can come and go when I'm between sales; I'm my own boss, and all the rest. Right! And yet here I am. I want to leave but I can't quite bring it together financially to do so. Sometimes I wonder when we will ever be together. We will, but the "when" is being incredibly elusive.

Dinner finds me at a friends this evening, instead of at McD's. It's a welcome relief complete with fine food and good company. And so ends another day.

Day 8. I'm still struggling like crazy. My money situation is bordering on the impossible! I try to ensure that it doesn't dominate my every thought but with each passing day it becomes harder and harder to ignore. I feel like such a loser right now. I still haven't paid my rent and everything that can be overdrawn has long since passed the friendly stage.

I really don't know what to do with this. I can't quit the one job that promises me the best way out of this mess. It's not like anyone is beating down my door to employ me at the moment. It's ironic when I think how most people see me: if I only had his skills and talents, if only . . . oh well, I clean up real good.

I'm not one to feel terribly sorry for myself but I'm a bit surprised at how few people have "stepped up" to offer any kind of assistance. Either they don't sense the need, or can't, or just don't believe me. Others, I'm sure, could care less. If I held a mirror up, I wonder which me I'd see? I must admit that I'm super sensitive at this moment so I may be misreading everyone's motives entirely.

I do have a few constants in my life. God, first and foremost. And Malena. Mom and McD's are right up there. Add in some incredible friends! These are my ports in the storm, and I am definitely in the eye of the hurricane right now. Sometimes I wonder if I will make it. There is so much against us and yet I'm convinced that we will prevail (convinced may be a little strong) if we continue to believe in each other and if indeed this is part of God's plan for our lives. We think it is.

But it's time to head back to McD's. I am struggling big time right now. Thank God I'm diarizing this journey or I'd probably be abandoning this project right about now!

Day 9. Yesterday was an absolute write off! Enough said!

Day 10. Tomorrow I weigh in and I'm expecting nothing short of a disaster! I need to at least get in one good day so here's hoping this is it! I am certainly a lot more fragile than I thought. I knew this would be difficult but it's even worse than I imagined.

But then the day began to change. The Pastor at the church I attend happened to be at McD's and mentioned that there was a symphony taking place at the church that evening.

I decided that I might as well attend. It was obvious that I needed to get around something positive because in the state I was in, I wasn't good for me or anybody else. Perhaps it was time to feed off of some positive energy and get the focus off myself for a bit.

During the intermission I scanned the crowd and it became obvious why I needed to be here. There he stood, alone, seemingly confused, and I knew I needed to speak to him. It was obvious that something was amiss, and as I approached, it became apparent that his wife was not with him. And that's when I found out that she had passed away a mere two months earlier.

I've learned that there are no words that are adequate at that time. I've learned that listening is what's required and I've become quite good at remembering that I have one mouth and two ears. And that's what was required.

And so a day that was going nowhere fast became a day that forced me to give the best of me. My silence was required and that I could deliver and it felt good.

WEIGH IN . . . Astoundingly, I lost 7.5 pounds! Maybe I can do this after all!

THE SECOND TEN DAYS - STAGE 1

Day 1. I finished up a real estate transaction this morning so now I'll head to Eaglesham to take my uncle shopping in Falher. I desperately need to get out of town for a while anyway.

That went well and I didn't overeat (I usually end up eating a burger, fries, and gravy when I go to Falher). Maybe I'm finally getting my act together! I stopped to visit my Mom at the Villa for a half hour or so and then I dropped in at my sister's place in Watino for a short visit. And then it was off to Eaglesham to drop off my uncle and have another short visit with some other good friends. Of course, short turned into a 2 hour visit.

DAY 2. Sunday, June 8/14. Time to head to church. Great message: 1. None are excluded, except by choice 2. None of us are perfect (I'm proof positive of that) 3. With God all things are possible.

Well, I had McD's for breakfast as usual and followed that up with lunch at Arby's and finished the evening munching on a bran muffin. What a disasterous week so far! But, I did finish the day off with a walk around the resevoir with a friend.

STRANGERS IN THE NIGHT

I decided that I needed to get some distance and some time away from Malena to figure out where this was going. I had promised myself that I would not get involved with anyone on this journey but of course, I did. And now I needed to think. So I left. For two months. And God did I miss her! Whether I liked it or not, this was very real and I needed to go back.

And go back I did! I wasn't sure what would happen the moment I opened that door; would we be two awkward strangers or . . . ?

But no. The moment our eyes met we knew that we were destined to be together. We knew there would be huge opposition but together we knew we were strong enough to survive anything that came our way. And trust me, there was a lot of opposition!

I stayed but 10 days on this trip but it would set the stage for our future together.

When I left on this journey of discovery months before, I knew not where I was going, or when, or even if I'd be coming back. I didn't really care one way or the other.

My family and friends were confused. They knew I was leaving but they certainly didn't know my state of mind. And then I came home. And I stayed for two months. Then I left again and went back to the same place. "We don't understand. We knew you wanted to travel, and we knew you had no set itinerary, but now you're back in Panama. What's going on? Don't tell us this is about a woman!" Oh dear. What else could it be possibly about?

And of course, they didn't understand. I didn't either. It wasn't like I didn't get "involved" from time to time, but this was different. I was in love and determined to change my life completely. I felt bad for all concerned but not bad enough that I would give up this exciting new life I was about to embark on. Not a chance! But then something happened that would change everything!

I was back in Canada working for a few months before heading down south again. I decided that since I was here anyway I might as well set up a Doctor's appointment. It had been a couple of years since I'd seen my Doctor so I figured the time was right. That decision probably saved my life!

DAY 3. Well, I'm down another pound but I'm not all that happy about it. 263.4 pounds this morning. I need to get exercising if I want to speed up this process and achieve some of the goals that I'd set for myself. Anyway, I'm off to McD's for a Bacon and Egg McGriddle and a Diet Coke. Love that stuff! I image that I'd make a lot more progress if I dumped the Diet Coke but I'm not quite ready to do that yet!

So, I headed over to the church to attend the CR program and of course, I had to eat first. And eat I did: lasagna, Caesar salad, and apple pie, and of course, a Diet Coke. It's only 6 pm so I think I'll be fine.

YOU CAN'T GO

I went to the Doctor, not because I felt anything was wrong, just that it was time. I knew I'd be leaving again soon, so why not?

"Have I seen you before?" He asked. "I'm pretty sure you have, yes." "I don't think so. Let me check. No, I haven't. We're going to do a full medical right now." Just like that. Wow. Wasn't expecting that!

And was he thorough! He probed everywhere but kept coming back to my chest area. Strange. I'd had the same Doctor for many, many years and I saw him regularly, but he certainly didn't check me out like this guy!

"Come with me." Ominous.

And out of his office we went, down the hall and into another Doctor's office. A heart specialist. Oh oh.

" I need you to listen to his heart, please." And she confirmed what he had already suspected. There was a slight murmur, barely detectable, but there nonetheless.

And that's when my life, once again, changed dramatically. Now there were some decisions to make.

It made no sense to me, especially now. I was about to embark on a whole new and exciting life that would take me far from the comforts of the existence I now knew.

But, confirmation was required, and I was booked within days to see a Cardiologist in Edmonton. I wouldn't be able to drive after the procedure so my daughters graciously agreed to drive, and besides, they could do a little shopping at West Edmonton Mall.

I didn't want them to be around when I got the results of the tests so I convinced them to go shopping and I'd contact them when I was done. Good thing. The results were anything but encouraging but I wasn't about to share that with them, at least not yet. I'm the type that needs to do some deep thinking and decide what information I would or would not share with anyone.

"I'm afraid we have bad news. You have severe aortic stenosis. It is extremely serious and we need to operate as soon as possible." What?

I stared at him but it was obvious that this was no joke. He continued "I don't understand how you had no symptoms. You said you had no shortage of breath, you weren't lethargic, or tired, you had no tightness in your chest, nothing at all to indicate a problem. That's very strange."

My God, I was on a volcano, I spent time in the sea, I spent lots of time in the jungle, I zip lined, I rappelled, I body surfed, and on and on and on. Obviously I got tired from time to time, but after all, I did a lot and I packed a few extra pounds that certainly weren't muscle! Of course that's tiring! And besides, most of the people I was doing all this stuff with were at least 20 years younger than me, so I thought nothing of it other than I'd better get back in shape real quick!

And now he wanted to rip my chest open. Forget that! I needed to think. I needed to get out of this hospital and do some research. And I told him so.

"And I need to go to Panama before I'll even consider this!" "You can't!" Oops! Bad choice of words. "Sorry Doctor, I'm not trying to be ignorant here but I have got to go back to Panama before I'll even consider surgery. You're talking open heart surgery, for God's sake!"

"I'll tell you what. Let's get you on the treadmill for a bit." And that's what we did. After a few minutes the cardiologist said "I can't stop you from going. You're incredibly healthy but you're not. I don't understand the lack of symptoms. The treadmill should have clarified a few things for us but it didn't. Please understand the risk that you're taking by delaying the surgery. You're strong right and that would help immeasurably with your recovery. If something happens in the meantime, it could end badly for you." I understood, but in my mind, I had no choice. I had to go to Panama and I had to decide whether I was going to let them rip my chest wide open!

My daughters kept asking what the prognosis was. I was so glad that I hadn't let them come in with me! "He says that they have some work to do on me but not right away. They'll get back to me with more details in the days ahead." I left it at that. I knew what everyone would say and how they would treat me once they knew. Forget that! I'm not an invalid and I don't want to treated as such. I didn't need everyone to be thinking that I could keel over at any moment. Of course, I didn't tell them what the Doctor had actually said. I didn't tell them that the term he used was "widow maker" and that it can happen without warning! "Don't you understand that the places you go, and the things you do are putting you in extreme danger!" Of course I did.

DAY 4. I got the results I deserved. No movement on the scale, again. This is not working well and yet, better habits are forming. I'm not eating after dinner anymore which is a bonus. I just need to get rid of that first 10 pounds! I'm going for a walk around the reservoir shortly with a good friend, I think. It's raining, but I love the rain!

So ends another day, and as usual, I was less than perfect. So here I sit in McDs writing these words that I now share with you. I know I'm making progress, albeit slowly. Moments ago, my phone rang, and it was my Doctor. I guess I have to see him again tomorrow. One step forward, two steps back. God, I hope not! I best not get ahead of myself.

Around 4 am I received a wonderful audio text from Malena. I awoke a few hours later to hear "Good morning Duane. I hope you have a great day! I love you." And that's why I will persevere despite the frustration. I just want to go home!

ROAD TRIP WITH MY GIRLS

So we made our plans for our road trip. What a great way to bond and share a unique experience with my daughters! "Dad, anywhere you want to go is fine with us." I wanted them to pick and choose and I would adapt as required. "OK. Vancouver Island, especially Victoria, if that's OK?" Of course it was, but it wasn't enough as far as I was concerned. "Where else do you want to go? There must be some place! What would you like to do" their typical answer: it's fun wherever you go so it doesn't really matter." At least they think I'm fun to be around! But I couldn't leave it there. So I introduced another element into the conversation to see where that would go, and boy, did I nail it!

"How about Port Angeles?"

Dead silence. "Hello?" "

"Did you say Port Angeles? Seriously?"

"Sure. Why not?"

"Oh my God, don't you know?"

"Know what?" Obviously I was missing something big time. A minute ago, they didn't care where they went and now . . .

"TWILIGHT".

"What's that supposed to mean?"

"Everyone knows about twilight!"

Obviously not everyone. So as we chatted, I googled Twilight and it all began to make sense. Well, sorta. The Twilight series of books that had sold millions of copies worldwide had been set in Port Angeles, Forks, LaPush, and so on, and now their Dad was telling them that they could go to this land of vampires and werewolves.

I had no idea how big a phenomena this was, but they soon educated me. And thus, our trip began to take shape. Washington state, particularly the Olympic Peninsula, would become the go to place in the days to come. I began learning about Edward, and Bella, as well as Jacob and the others, much more than I ever needed or wanted to know. The fait accompli was spending a couple of nights in a blood themed room adorned with the photos of the aforementioned characters which were now dominating our lives. But, I absolutely refused to go vampire and werewolf hunting. That they could do on their own!

As distracted as they were about this journey, they were still unsure of exactly what their Dad was telling them about his "visit" with the Cardiologist. Apparently I have a habit of minimizing issues from time to time, and this is one that definitely fit in that category. "It's not fair that we don't know!"

So I told them most of it. Except for the part about the Doctor wanting me to be available immediately for open heart surgery. After all, we had planned this road trip and I wasn't about to cancel it just because the Doctors were freaking out! That seemed to settle the issue, at least for now, so enough said. Oh, and I conveniently failed to mention to them the email I had just received that morning informing me that a bed was available to me 5 days from now would not be used by me. I know this sounds incredibly arrogant, but I had things to do and people to see first. It was a chance I was prepared to take!

So we journeyed for two weeks. I felt this would be a wonderful bonding opportunity and it certainly was. After all, I knew my life was going to change in a huge way, and I wasn't talking about the "heart thing" either. My next flight, only days away, would take me to Panama, where I would have to tell Malena exactly what we were up against, and THAT I wasn't looking forward to!

FACE TO FACE

She knew something was up and that it was serious. And though she was excited that I was coming, she was afraid. What was it that I wouldn't tell her over the phone?

I knew it would be tough but I needed to do it, and in person. So I did, but there is no gentle way to break that kind of news. She was afraid. She was happy that I was there but angry that I had come. "You should be in the hospital! What if something happens to you down here?" I knew she was right but it mattered not. I needed to see her; I needed to tell her in person. Most would think that the decision to go to Panama was foolish, and perhaps it was, but I could not bring myself to tell her except in person. I was very aware that once I went under the knife that I may never see her again. I had to prepare her for whatever may happen, and I knew I had to see her before I would consent to the inevitable. And now I had. So now I would do what had to be done.

I am a person of faith, and anyone who walked in the shoes I had these past months, would understand the position I had taken. Nothing in my world happened by coincidence, of that I am convinced, and the very narrow road I had found myself on had led me straight to her. I tried to deny it for a time. The whole situation bordered on the impossible, even for me, and yet I knew in my heart of hearts that God was mixed up in this somehow!

We knew it would be tough. Open heart surgery is definitely not a walk in the park! Recovery times are unpredictable. Depression can rear its' ugly head; get up and go often takes a hike. And, Malena was 6000+ miles away (10,000 km). My people knew little of her. Communication between them would be awkward at best, and yet, if I was going under the knife, communicate they must!

Day 5. I'm not getting the results I desire. I wonder if it's because I'm not doing my part? You think? At this juncture I am losing around .6 pounds daily. In someone else's world that may be fine. In mine, it's not!

I AM NOT AFRAID

Malena was scared. Here I was telling her that they were going to split me open but not to worry. We had known each other for such a short time, and yet it felt like we'd known each other for years. She couldn't contain her fear, and strange though it was, I was more concerned for her than for myself. I comforted her as best I could; I talked about our great health care system; and I told her how the Doctors had said what great shape I was in and that I would get through this with flying colours. I told her all this stuff, and I told myself the same story, but at the end of the day, they were still going to crack me open, and that was a fact!

I've been asked by many of the people I knew well whether I was afraid or not. I found that to be an interesting question. So many others who had went through open heart surgery, and these were people of supposed deep faith, told me how afraid they had been. I found that somewhat perplexing.

So why wasn't I afraid? I kept asking myself that question. I was calm, unafraid, and resolved to do what must be done. I had done my research; I had presented the Doctor with the best body I could at the time; we had discussed the various options and settled on what was the most appropriate for me. I felt that I had the right surgeon, and logically, considering the relationship I was involved in, it made no sense that the outcome would be anything but good. And last, but certainly not least, I knew God was with me all the way! I was, and still am, convinced that Malena and I would have never crossed paths without divine intervention. Many will use a couple of "coincidences" to make a case for or against something. Try 20 or 30 so called "coincidences" and then tell me what you think! I think God has plans to keep me working for at least 40 more years! I have to say though, I was never afraid. Never.

I promised her that I would be back in a few short months, that we would be together. Have faith! And then I told her that she'd have to speak to my daughters before I went into surgery. And again, after I came out of it. That scared her, and it scared my daughters, but it was something they'd have to do.

DAY 6. Thursday June 12. Time to head to the Doctors' appointment. I know that something is not quite right, and unfortunately, I was right. At least now we know what we have to deal with. I bet I start losing weight a lot faster from here on in. Enough about this for now. I'm dragging my butt these days and my mind is going along for the ride. The only satisfaction I'm getting from this journey at the moment is strictly from being available to help, or at least being available to listen to those who need an ear. That I can do. I'm feeling totally inadequate, and I might add, impotent at the moment. This has been going on far too long! I'm so lonely right now!

AND NOW I LIVE

So I made the call. "Hi hon. I have the girls with me. I need you to talk to each other." The fear on the other end of the phone was palpable. She knew this was coming . She knew she would be eventually meeting my kids, but she never envisioned it being in these kinds of circumstances! She was so afraid that they wouldn't like her, wouldn't accept her, and yet, she knew that wasn't true. They had sent her a card on one of my excursions down there, and the contents of that card had blown her away! In fact, they conveyed to her that they very much looked for-ward to meeting her, and her kids in the future. I remember how overwhelmed she was with their support for the two of us. "We just want our Dad to be happy." But this was different. And this was now.

When I handed the phone to the girls they were as terrified as she. They wanted to get to know her as well, but not like this!

But, if you know me at all, you knew that they were going to be talking, and they were going to be talking now!

And talk they did. First one daughter, then the other. This had to happen tonight because tomorrow morning they were going to split me open. There were no guarantees and I needed them to step up to the plate. Hopefully, the call they would make tomorrow would be a good news call, but regardless, the call had to be made and it was up to them.

It was time, and of course, the date is registered in my mind: Oct 11, 2011. I knew I was supposed to be worried , even afraid, but I wasn't. I had done all that I could do. It was out of my hands now and it was up to the surgeon to do his thing. I trusted him, and I trusted that God wanted me around a bit longer. After all, I had taken on a huge amount of responsibility in a land far removed from my birth, and I'm convinced He was instrumental in all that had taken place in Panama!

Just having what I suspected, confirmed, gave me hope. Something could be done about this and I think it was interfering with my weight loss, my mood, and definitely my energy. It was time to put the excuses away, even the so called good ones.

I mentioned to the surgeon that my daughters were here, and that they would be the contacts for all those who were waiting to hear the outcome of my operation. I lamented the fact that Malena couldn't be here, that she was 6000 miles away, and how I wished I could hear her voice when I woke up. "Duane, I'll make it happen."

The operation was a success and the girls made the appropriate calls to spread the word. And of course, they called Malena. When I came to that evening, she was allowed to speak to me, though I heard not the words. That didn't matter. It was the point of it. I asked her later if I had made any sense when we were talking and she assured me that indeed, I had! And though we were thousands of miles apart, we were together. I knew it going into the operation, and I knew it when I awoke.

DAY 7. 263.4. I'm reasonably happy with my results considering that I've been somewhat absent this whole time. I woke up feeling different this morning. More determined, I think. I hope.

DAY 8. The weight loss numbers refuse to move, and yet I know that I'm beginning to win the battle. It seems that about .5 pounds is what I'm ending up with. I guess I should be happy about this, after all, if I can lose 15 pounds in a month I should be ecstatic, right? Not only will my health improve dramatically, but I'll look a heck of a lot better too! I know that sounds rather egotistical but hey, I'm human you know!

I'm in my office again this evening, alone as usual. It never used to bother me much, but the longer we are apart, the lonelier I get. Even so, we are stronger and more resolved than ever. Our time is coming, and one day soon, I will go home to be with her! In the meantime, I'll continue to do what can only be done here, and fight the weight battle at the same time!

The evenings are always the toughest. I've had enough sustenance for the day but emotionally I'm drained.

I had hoped a solution to a "temporary" problem would reveal itself tonight but it didn't. So as a result I'm a bit stressed out. Sure hope I don't use that as an excuse to pig out! I know. More water. And a banana.

DAY 9. Progress! 261 pounds this morning! 11 pounds gone! Less than I should have shed in the past 18 days in my opinion but still significant. So I'll take the victory and be glad for it.

It seems like my life consists of work, church, McD's, and a few meetings every week. When I say it that way, it seems rather normal. Oh yeah, Malena is only 6000 miles away! Normal, indeed!

McD's has served me well. It's my refuge, my meeting place, my writing place, and lest we forget, my eating place. I know I've abused that last one in the past but that was then. It's different now. I hope.

I'm leaving in a few months, and that is a fact! And I hope to take a lot less of me on the next trip!

Day 10. Monday. 261.2 pounds. Gotta like that! Blood Pressure 125/69. Wow! Work is a struggle right now. I have interested buyers but no one is pulling the trigger. It's frustrating and fear is definitely stronger than faith at this moment. I am literally down to my last buck and I don't know where to go from here. Lord, please help me! I'm trying so hard to let go and let God.

When I get to this point I have to be really diligent and not give in and just eat to feel better, even though I know I'll feel worse later. Still, I ended up eating 2 Bacon and Egg McGriddles, a bran muffin, and a copious amount of Diet Coke. A bit later I added in 2 burgers, a bunch of cheddar, a quantity of veggies, and more pop. Yea, me!

And then a call came along with an offer I couldn't refuse. How can I not look upward? Maybe, just maybe, I'm beginning to get it!

Verdict: I'm now down 12 pounds . . . Yes!

FLASHBACK

When I arrived in Panama three months after my open heart surgery, I was pretty excited. I knew I had come through the surgery with flying colours, and now I could spend the next month with Malena before heading back to Canada to work. And though she was happy to see me, she was shocked at how "skinny" I was! Trust me, I was not skinny, but she was used to seeing me quite another way! "Please don't lose any more weight. You're a big guy. I like you that way!"

Go figure! I had to laugh when she called me skinny. I don't think I've ever been called that, at least not in a very long time! But, she was serious. So, I had to use another approach. "I need to do this for health reasons. You do want me around for a long time, don't you?" What could she say? "Yes, of course." Does she really think I'd do this just for vanity reasons? Interesting. I mean, it is for health reasons, of course, but I admit, I do want to look as good as I can. Not because I'm insecure or anything, or looking around, I just like to feel good about myself. I admit, looking good certainly helps the self-esteem! She certainly didn't have to worry about me snooping around. She and I were connected by a lot more than words, and though we had known each other for a relatively short time, we were a couple and determined to stay that way despite the many forces that would seek to tear us apart!

THE THIRD TEN DAYS - STAGE 1

Day 1. And now 20 days are gone! I accomplished something despite my best effort to self sabotage. I'm averaging .6 pounds per day and I'm beginning to believe in myself a little bit more each day.

Of course I had a McGriddle this morning as well as one burrito. The afternoon found me here once more chowing down on a bran muffin, and later I finished off the day with a Sweet Chili McWrap. As you can see, my love affair with McD's still continues! And of course, I had copious amounts of Diet Coke throughout the day.

WE WILL NOT BE DENIED

I spent a wonderful month with Malena but, all too soon, it was time to go. I admit, her life is a lot less complicated when I'm not around. Not everyone is on board with our relationship but we are determined to make it work. We both want it and we're both prepared to make whatever sacrifices that are necessary to sustain it.

This would prove to be much more of a challenge than I could have ever imagined. I thought I'd be able to head south every 2-3 months but economics raised its ugly head time and time again. I couldn't understand why I wasn't performing up to par. I was falling short of my goals, and even though we were doing incredibly well considering all the obstacles in our path, seeing her every 5-6 months was not something I thought I could ever live with. In days past, I know for a fact that I couldn't have survived that type of a relationship. But, for some reason, this was different and I wasn't about to let it go. Not a chance! And neither was she! Together we knew we could do this. We had to keep our eyes on the goal line. We would be together one day. And she constantly reminded me "we are together, we're just not in the same place, not yet. Don't stress over it or soon you will give up on us. I'm not giving up! Don't you!"

I won't.

Though we fight tooth and nail for this relationship, I find myself alone a lot. I'm actually pretty good at being alone, but there are times when it is extremely difficult. I don't want to compromise myself in any way so I fill my time working, of course, and spending as much time as I can with friends, and friends yet unmade, church functions, writing groups, and so on. And of course, I spend an inordinate amount of time at McD's writing my next award winning novel. Uh huh!

Although I spend a lot of time in McD's and I eat here exclusively (almost), I still try to eat moderately. Of course, I've abused that in the past, and as a result, I find myself on this quest to lose weight once again. I had allowed myself to get quite heavy once again and ultimately settled in around the 250 pound mark. Remember, she liked me right where I was at, but

I didn't. I was becoming lethargic. I knew the situation we found ourselves it was adding to the depression I was feeling, and I knew I had to get my act together, and quickly. So I went to the Doctor. There was nothing clinically wrong, as I suspected, but I had to do something. The next trip saw me arrive in Panama around the 260 pound mark, and incredibly unhappy. Malena didn't seem to mind but she knew it was bothering me. When I'm there, I lose weight. She cooks sparingly, fast food is out, and I'm where I want to be. Add in the heat factor and it's a no brainer!

Work is slow for me. I'm anxious and that usually leads me to eating as a form of escape. I want to go home and I can't. I'm not a happy camper right now! We seem to be getting farther apart, and with each passing day, I'm gaining a bit more weight. And that's why, 21 days ago, I said enough is enough! The scales shocked me: 272 pounds! I had to get it together, and it had to be now! As you can tell, the first few days were a write off but slowly I started to get my act together. I couldn't quit. If I did, I was done, and so were we! So I sucked it up and I started getting results, and now I'm a believer. I want this real bad!

Day 2. And now I'm down 14 pounds! If I ramp this up a bit and start exercising I might just pull this off!

I'm in a strange space at the moment, and the landscape is in a state of flux. Big, big decisions await my execution and I'm about to make them. Not everyone will be happy, but such is life. This is an exciting time, and though stressful, my eye is definitely on the goal line. Most of you know of what I speak, and for those who don't, soon you will.

So I came back from Panama determined to not only never gain back any of that extra weight, but to continue on the journey to even better health, but, it didn't quite work out that way and over the following months I think I became despondent and wondered when we would ever be able to pull this thing together properly. I wanted to be in Panama but I was stuck here. Bad decisions in the past would rear their ugly head and I would find myself repeating many of the behaviours of the past.

Just because one knows better doesn't mean that one won't repeat yesterday. That became abundantly obvious! It's quite fine to eat at McD's as much as I do (ok, it's not), as long as I'm not overdoing it, but it provided a semblance of comfort that I sorely needed. It was easy to justify, after all, there were a lot worse things I could be doing. And that was true of course, but I soon began paying a price for my reliance on my chosen menu.

I guess I must have believed Malena about being "too skinny" because over the next couple of months I gained back at least 15 pounds. These weren't healthy pounds either. The Doctor was emphatic about continuing to lose weight and maintain the lifestyle that I had prior to the surgery. Yes, I was heavier than I should have been, but I was in pretty good shape, and now I was heading down a one way street going the wrong way!

I couldn't understand me! Didn't I want what I said I wanted? She was waiting for me in Panama. Yet, here I was, self-sabotaging at every opportunity!

Day 3. 258.4. Friday. BP 130/80. I thought I should have lost a bit more weight but I know better than to expect movement on the scale on a daily basis. I'm heading out on a road trip today and I know that will cause some diet issues! I am so weak!

Day 4. Not sure how well I'm doing. Can't check the scales, and even though I'm being good, I did have a couple slices of a meat eaters pizza. I think I made it through the day ok but I can't jump on the scales until Sunday. Oh boy!

Day 5. I'm in Watino, for the burial of my uncle's ashes. I knew this would be a tough day. There would be an abundance of homemade food, and I am weak. Besides, I rarely get any home cooking so it's a disaster waiting to happen! I did weaken, not a lot, but enough that I knew the consequences would show up on the scales. If I'm to be successful in this endeavour, I absolutely, positively, must not eat at night! But, eat at night I did!

Day 6. Sunday, June 22. 263.8 I definitely tested the scales this morning. When this happens, it would be so easy to just say forget it. I won't, but I want to. So, it's back to McD's for a little portion control this morning. A McGriddle and Diet Coke would have to do.

And I'm off to church. It was a typical great message followed by a terrific lunch which challenged my resolve yet again.

So now I write and my mind plays tricks on me. Eat, eat, eat, after all, you deserve it! Yeah, right! I'm kind of down on myself right now. I keep blowing it. And my mind wanders to Panama and that is always dangerous. But, and there's always a but, I did go for a long walk around the college with a good friend.

I decided to go to a movie this evening and I almost talked myself out of the popcorn, but I didn't. So a tub of popcorn loaded with butter made it onto the menu.

I had better get this figured out real quick. Days are passing and I'm going backwards.

Panama is where my heart is and I am determined to be there with her. And though I say this, I don't appear to be backing it up with the action steps that are required. I am working but the results are not forthcoming. That is confusing to me. I don't usually have an earning problem, just a spending problem. That's bad enough, but put the two together and it's a disaster!

Day 7. 261 pounds. BP 149/83. What a blessing to wake up this morning and be able to hear properly! It's been a long time. I've struggled with hearing loss in my right ear for 3 years.

The hearing clinic was puzzled as well; their tests indicated that all was well, and yet it wasn't. The Ear, Nose, and Throat Specialist figured a few steroids should clear whatever was ailing. Nothing. Back and forth. I knew I couldn't settle for this; I knew something could be done and still I let it go. One year, two, and finally, in frustration I went to my Doctor once again. He referred me to another specialist and this time results would be different.

My Dad was virtually deaf and I remember how it robbed him of so much quality of life. It frustrated him to no end to sit among a group and be unable to participate in a conversation. Eventually he would avoid crowds altogether, and engage in only one on one conversations. Soon he began to isolate himself further and further. Sad but true. I knew that I was getting a taste of what he experienced on a daily basis, and I knew I had to insist on getting this problem rectified.

The night before I saw the next specialist an amazing thing happened. I was laying in bed when my ear suddenly started to drain. That had happened before, but within seconds, I would be deaf again, and no matter what I did, I could never get my hearing back except for a few seconds at a time. Except this time, it was different. I was hearing when I went to sleep and I was hearing when I woke up. Oh my God! And to top it off, today I'd be seeing the specialist. This should be interesting!

This Specialist was on the ball and one prescription later, along with a few instructions and I was on my way. It seems I had swimmers ear that hadn't been diagnosed properly and that an infection had established itself and wasn't about to let go. Until the previous night.

Malena was unimpressed. She had come up with that diagnoses 2 years before, simply by smelling my ear. Better medical care in Canada, you say? Right!

I must say that I'm feeling pretty good right about now! Ears that hear, and eyes that see should never be taken for granted. Nothing in our lives should be, but often we do. I so much want to live the life I believe I've been created for, to live out my purpose. I believe I have a handle on where God is leading me, and it is imperative that I continue to work on this temple so that I may endure, that I may run the good race, and that I cross the finish line according to His purpose.

Day 8. More of the same. I've got to watch the head games so I don't fall into my usual trap. I'm going to have to keep busy today or I'll blow it. Time to head to the trails for a walk. I usually have no problem throwing down a few words but today I'm struggling. I guess I'll have to settle for "less is more" on this day.

Day 9. 260.6 pounds. It's pretty obvious that I have to pump up the volume if I'm going to achieve the results that I want. Two thirds of this first month are nearly gone. I was expecting great things from myself and I'm not sure that I'm delivering the goods. The next while should be very interesting!

I've tried to do this while maintaining an almost intimate relationship with McDonald's. I refuse to abandon McD's as it is important to me for a lot of reasons. I must admit, that to an outsider, this must seem ridiculous, but I assure you, it is not! When I think about the countless relationships that would not have existed had I chosen another venue, it becomes mind boggling! I've made myself open and available to whomever desired to spend some time with me. That has been many, many people over the years. I decided to really open my eyes and look far beyond myself, and as a result, I've really learned to "see" other people. With great regularity they approach me. Perhaps it is merely a coffee but often it is a great deal more. We, as a society, are an incredibly lonely bunch, and when someone pays attention to us, we respond in kind. I believe this is part of my mission and I fully intend to fulfil my purpose.

Day 10. 259 this am. "It don't come easy. Gotta pay your dues if you want to sing the blues . . . it don't come easy." So said Ringo Starr so long ago. That's how I feel about this attempt of mine to lose a pile of weight. "It don't come easy." But then, why should it? I certainly did my part piling the excess on, and now I must labor, and deservedly so!

It is such an incredible feeling to hear again! The past three years have been extremely frustrating in so many ways, and having an ear that refused to hear merely added to the misery that already was. Three days have now passed and I'm hearing perfectly again! Dare I hope! I've been fortunate in my life to escape, at least to this point, many of the infirmaries that seem to incapacitate so many people. So, I will keep my whining to a minimum, and on the occasion that I do, I will have a little cheese with it. Of course, knowing me, I'll probably gain some weight! In any case, the first 30 days are nearly over. My mind continues to play games with me. But, this is a battle I must win. I will endure, and I will finish this race in fine style! I will!

VERDICT

Final results after 30 days: 15 pounds are gone! I'm averaging .5 pounds per day, with 10 days to go in the first 40 day challenge.

THE FOURTH 10 DAYS - STAGE 1

Day 1. So I'm down to 257 pounds. I'm still averaging .5 pounds per day so I'm certainly on track. Yes! I dropped off some friends at the airport a few minutes ago so now it's time to head over to McD's for a Bacon and Egg McGriddle and a Diet Coke. I would have much rather be winging my way south but I guess I'll have to settle for breakfast.

This promises to be another busy day. I have a showing around noon and an inspection set up for 3pm. I'm also awaiting a removal of conditions on another property, and that all important call from Panama.

The inspection was a bust! Back to the drawing board. So now I'm at the office setting up a few showings for tomorrow.

And then it was off to dinner with a friend, which incredibly, I didn't screw up! My diet is intact and all is right with the world.

Day 2. I'm up early today. I feel the energy coming back and I'm becoming a believer. In me. But it's time to head to McD's once again. I crave this place, especially at breakfast, and today would be no different. I'm incredibly loyal to this particular McD's. I wonder if it's because of the star treatment I always receive here?

Since I began this odyssey a month ago, I haven't stumbled much at all, after the first week, surprisingly. I remember how hard it was just to make the commitment aloud, actually saying to myself "I will do this!" And then the disaster of the first week and yet I decided "to tell all" and stick it out regardless of whether I succeeded or failed. That was scary. Ironically, I need McD's at this time. It helps me portion control as well as providing numerous other benefits. But the one thing this has taught me is this: no night eating after 6 pm! Whatever it is I'm doing is working and I'll stick with it to the end of this challenge!

I've been looking back over the past 32 days. I started this challenge on May 28/14. I didn't want to, but desperation forced me to go on record each day regardless of whether it was good, bad, or ugly! I must admit that I now look forward to each passing day knowing that I am closer and closer to achieving my goal!

Day 3. Wow! I'm down 17 pounds now! The rain is coming down and I'm loving it! Of course, McD's has my attention again this morning and a McGriddle and Diet Coke await me, so I've got to go! Darn, I'm still hungry so I followed up with a breakfast burrito. Gotta love it!

I loved the church service today. The pastor spoke on baptism and issued a challenge to those in the audience.

"If you have't been baptized and you want to, why not do it now?" And with that challenge put forth, 14 people stepped forward, street clothes and all. We're talking full immersion here. But come they did anyway. And away they went, soaking wet but incredibly happy!

I worked part of the day and then spent some time with a great friend discussing the wonderful world of the would be writer. I have no doubt that some of us will move on to share our words with the world. Maybe even me!

Day 4. I was hoping to do a bit better than I'm doing but I know I should be happy with the results I'm getting. I know I'm impatient. I know it took a long time to put the weight on but still . . . I've started throwing my work out clothes in the vehicle just in case I get ambitious. I know exercise is vital if I want to maintain or make this loss permanent. In the past, the closer I got to my goal the more I picked up the pace. I'm hoping that that happens again!

Time to head to McD's. I need my Bacon and Egg McGriddle and Diet Coke to kick off my day. It's only 7 am but I'm feeling good. I have a busy day ahead of me but that's exactly how I like it!

Lunch consisted of a Sweet Chili McWrap and of course, a Diet Coke. I know I need to make a few changes to my menu but that ain't gonna happen today!

CR tonight. It's a program sponsored by the church I attend. Plus, they put on an awesome dinner at a very reasonable cost. The only problem is that I can't or won't portion control, so I'll resist it once again and head to McD's for dinner. I'm eating smaller dinner portions now so a McDouble, small fries, and Diet Coke would serve as my dinner this evening. But at least I portion controlled!

And for the critics among you, know this: it's all about control at this juncture for me. I don't trust myself enough to stray from that which is working for me. I try to stay out of precarious situations, at least for the time being. I know this has to change, and it will in due course. For now, this works. Enough said!

Day 5. 252.8 pounds. BP 144/80. Canada Day. It's all coming together at last. But still, I need breakfast and McD's is my standby. And then I decided to take a road trip to Eaglesham which is a couple of hours away from here. Needless to say, the parade and celebration in a small town is rather different than that at Grande Prairie.

But, I had a job to do, and with the recruitment of one other fellow, we hauled a bed up to my uncles. My Mom is moving into a villa and it was my job to arrange the bed move. Of course, I knew there would be a problem on this day. There is no McD's here, so I headed to the Eaglesham fairgrounds to partake in whatever morsels I could find. Wouldn't you know it: there was a cheeseburger just waiting there with my name on it. I wanted another but managed to resist. So far, so good.

At least the bed had made its move and I decided to head back to Grande Prairie and the sanctuary of my McD's. A McDouble, small fries, and Diet Coke put me into a happy place and I escaped this day relatively unscathed.

I know I can't continue down this path forever and continue to lose weight but for now I feel I have little choice. 19.2 pounds lost is pretty darn good considering that I'm somewhat of a loose cannon right now.

Day 6. Stayed the same as yesterday but I'm not complaining. I'm pumped and I'm determined to turn up the volume a bit more. If I can do this 10 days at a time I should be able to lose the 40 pounds. That's my initial goal and I'm determined to do it, hopefully in 80 days or so. Of course, I'm writing this from McD's where I just had another Bacon and Egg McGriddle as well as a breakfast burrito and my ever present Diet Coke. If I can stick with the portions ritually it is proving to not be terribly difficult. At least today. And as long as I don't eat at night.

A friend suggested that I include my daily menus in the back of this book to remove any doubt about my consumption. And that's why you won't see me include every item that I've eaten in the main text. I assure you, nothing has been added that I didn't actually eat but I may have forgot to include the odd cheezie binge!

I am certainly not advocating that anyone should follow my menu. Do so at your own peril, but this is what I did and these are the results I got.

And then it was off to Tony Roma's for dinner, and for the first time since I started this odyssey, I actually had a salad (Asian with grilled chicken). And it was delicious! So, I'm not addicted to McD's as you may have thought, but I need McD's as my control centre, and that will continue as long as I think it's required.

I wish I could say that I've been exercising regularly but I haven't. I can't seem to find the gear necessary to take this to the next level. In the past, exercise was the key to accomplishing my goals and now I'm incredibly lethargic. Today was the exception and I racked up several miles this afternoon. Maybe, just maybe! Boy, was I tired after that! I've got to get it going, and soon!

One more trip to McD's before the day is done. I decided that a bran muffin and Diet Coke would have to do, and that's the way it ended on this day. One day I will divorce the Diet Coke but that may be a ways off yet!

Day 7. I finally did it! 20.2 pounds are officially gone! I celebrate by heading to McD's and eating my usual McGriddle, a breakfast burrito, and several Diet Coke.

I can tell this is going to be a trying day. I want to celebrate my success but the problem is that I want to celebrate it by eating. So I headed over to the church for lunch today and I must say, I did ok. A grilled cheese sandwich, a couple of pickles and a Diet Coke took care of the cravings. So far, so good.

It may appear that I'm thumbing my nose at convention but that is not the case. As I've said repeatedly, this is what is working for me at this juncture. I am well aware that I will need to buckle down and change a few eating habits along the way if I wish to continue making progress. I believe I'm already making subtle changes, and I will continue to record these as I make the changes.

I have said repeatedly that I need to pick up the exercise quotient substantially, and I know it needs to begin "now." I am at a loss why this is taking me so long to "get into."

As I approach the end of the first 40 days, it is with trepidation and anticipation all rolled into one. You see, I've set my goal to lose 40 pounds, hopefully within 3 months, but I've just realized that the number 40 was even more significant than I first realized. When I recovered from the open heart surgery and then got the A-OK from my Doctor to fly, fly away, the scales announced a weight of 233 pounds. It had been many years since I'd seen that number and it was imperative that I use this number as a starting point to get my weight down to the 200-205 pound range. That had always been my sweet spot, that place where I was incredibly fit and incredibly strong. I was lean, I was fast, and I had energy to spare. Nothing could defeat me, at least in my minds' eye. That was a long time ago, and even though I gained a substantial amount of weight I was always in pretty good condition. But that was then, and this is now. If I want to live a long, healthy life, I need to get it together.

So I just realized that the 40 pound goal I had set for myself would put me at 232 pounds, 1 pound less than after the surgery. And that would become my new starting point. Coincidence? Probably, but I'll use it to my advantage. Now the number 40 has taken on a new significance. It's somewhat depressing to know that my journey, even upon losing the 40 pounds, will still have a long way to go but I'll take the victory for what it is.

As I stated earlier, when I arrived in Panama at a weight of 233 pounds, Malena thought I was "too skinny". Go figure! But, of course, she realized that from a health perspective I needed to lose even more weight. I had to laugh. The last time I'd been called skinny? Never!

I looked good and I felt great, at least in my opinion. And Malena's "too skinny" comment made me feel even better! But of course, I had to keep my health front and centre so Malena said she would certainly do her part. No McDs, no Pop, especially Diet Coke, and minimalist meals would be in order. Yes ma'am. And I did pretty good the month I was there, but all too soon it was time to return to Canada, and unfortunately, to the long formed habits of yesterday.

Day 8. 251.8 pounds. After everything I consumed yesterday, I feel quite fortunate to have stayed the same. So today I will bear down and get back on track. I know I need to be disciplined if I want to achieve my goals. Of course, I'm at McD's writing this while consuming a McGriddle and of course, Diet Coke. Sorry Malena!

The kind of work I do can be frustrating at times. Hurry up. Wait. Wait some more. I know the Mortgage Broker will call when they have the necessary approvals in place. Hopefully soon. Guess I'll just wait to hear.

I met some friends for lunch at, oh yeah, McD's. A McDouble, small fries, and Diet Coke once again made up my menu. I've been doing pretty well but I'm being a little nonchalant and that can bite me in the butt.

I'm already thinking of the next 10 days but I'd better get my mind on completing this 10 day stint first of all. And I've got to start exercising something besides my elbow at the dinner table!

When I allow myself, I start to get excited about the possibilities. 20 pounds is 20 pounds and I need to acknowledge that and give myself some credit for hanging in there. I can't continue to beat up on myself because that just takes me to a dark place.

I finished off the evening by taking in a movie complete with buttered popcorn and pop. At least it was a medium popcorn! And then I went for a stroll in the park with a friend. All is not lost.

Day 9. July 5/14. I'm staying the same, much to my chagrin, yet I have no one to blame but myself. My head loves playing games.

I had my usual breakfast at McD's and then I hit the trails with a vengeance before returning to McDs for a bran muffin and a pop. If you ever want to find me, you know where to look!

I walked around the reservoir twice today. I think I've got this finally. And then I returned to you know where to write and to dine. The Sweet Chili McWrap is oh so good! And that's a wrap for today. For the rest of the evening the only item on the menu is water.

I've long stated how important McD's is to me. It certainly isn't just about the food. I'm comfortable here. There's plenty of seating, the wifi works fine, and there is an ever changing sea of humanity that is representative of the world at large. I like that. It gives me energy and it helps me keep focused on my long term goals.

A great many people will be angry that I would dare to find the positive in a place like this. After all, these places are killing us with unhealthy food, and you extol their virtues? How dare you?

My response "Go somewhere else, and take your attitude with you."

Some of you would never darken the doorway of such places. Perfect! Then we don't have to put up with your superior attitudes. We all win! As for me and my kind, these establishments are more than a place to eat; they serve as microcosms that invite us into the lives of people that come from all over the world. And for that, I am truly grateful.

As well, I've gotten to know many of the staff here; I get to know about their lives, their countries, their sacrifices, their goals, and their dreams. I get to know them as real people and I love it! Plus, it helps me cope with the loneliness I experience by being so far away from my family. 6000 miles and months of separation are difficult to maintain. These people give me an incredible amount of strength as my situation, though extreme, pales in comparison to the sacrifices many of them make on a daily basis. So many of them have left husbands, or wives, and most have left children back home for the opportunity to better their lives. I love these people!

Day 10. Only 1 day remains in the first 40 days so it's best I don't blow it. The big weigh in is tomorrow. Of course, I am writing this from my barstool at my favourite watering hole. I couldn't resist having a McGriddle as well as a breakfast burrito and Diet Coke.

It's off to church for me and then back to McD's for a pop and bran muffin. And then it's time to hit the trails once again. My kids called and wanted to meet at Arby's. When I'm around food I can't seem to resist, so I had a roast beef sandwich and a pop. I'd better watch my eating the rest of the day or I'll blow the weigh-in tomorrow.

I decided to take in a movie this evening. The Tom Cruise flick, The Edge of Tomorrow got my attention. I resisted the popcorn this time and hopefully I can resist any temptation the rest of this day.

It's pretty apparent that I eat whatever I want and that at least 90% of the time that takes place at McD's. It works for me, and even though I know I could probably have done better eating elsewhere, I seem to need this place right now. It's working, and as long as it is, I'm staying here.

40 DAYS LATER

I'm down 20.2 pounds, slightly over .5 pounds daily through the first 40 days. It took me a while to get traction, but I did eventually. I really expected better results than this when I first began, but have since realized what a victory I've achieved. 40 days and 20 pounds gone! What's not to like?

I didn't set out to scoff at convention. I'm very serious about getting back in shape. I just knew that McDs satisfied me on many levels and I wasn't about to compromise that just yet. I'm stronger now, by far, than I was 40 days ago. I now know that I can do this. I'm going all the way. As long as I stay out of my own way.

I hope you've found my story to this point somewhat interesting; perhaps it's your story too. I've been frustrated, depressed, hopeless at times, and yet at other times, hopeful, euphoric, and excited by life's possibilities!

LETS BEGIN . . . AGAIN

Day 1. So I begin day 41 at 251.8 pounds. I'm reasonably happy but determined to do even better over the next 10 days. Time will tell. I know that normally weight loss gets more difficult as time goes on, but I'm incredibly motivated by my previous success so hopefully I can build on that.

I'm trying not to project too far ahead but that is proving difficult to do. I want this. I want to experience that 40 pound loss mark, and then the 50, and dare I say it, the 60 pound and beyond loss, which translates into winner, winner, winner! I want this badly!

I know that many of you disagree with my methodology, and that is your right, but I've stated emphatically over and over that this is what is working for me. Not once have I suggested that you should do the same. This is working for me and that's why I'm doing it.

Well, another deal crashed and burned this afternoon. When will I be smart enough to get out of this business? I think I'd better look up "insanity" again!

Headed to McD's for lunch again today and had all the usual gastronomic delights. I can tell I'm frustrated. I want to chow down. I know that is not a solution but that's what I want to do!

I should have headed to the park to blow off some steam but, of course, I didn't! That would have been way too sensible!

It's off to CR for me, and wouldn't it be like Shaun to serve turkey, mashed potatoes, gravy, beans, salads, and desert. And I indulged. Yes I did. It was good and I was weak and there you have it!

I've been pretty focused except for today so I'm going to cut myself a little slack. Yeah, I screwed up a bit. So what? Tomorrow is a new day.

Day 2. I got lucky. I stayed the same despite my collapse yesterday. Now it's time to regroup once again. Of course, I'm writing this at McD's where I just had a Bacon and Egg McGriddle and large Diet Coke!

GONNA CLIMB THAT MOUNTAIN

I'm stopping at the office for a bit and then heading to the trails. It's time to pick up the volume and I am definitely ready. I'm having a hard time understanding what's going on in my life right now. So much of it is great, and then I get sucker punched.

So, either I can sit here and whine about the inequities of life, or I can do something about it. I think that perhaps I will go with the latter, but first, I have something to do. A couple of phone calls and I have some company and I'm on my way. I'm off to Dunvegan. I have a huge climb in front of me and I am determined that today will be the day that I conquer the hill once more. I've dropped over 20 pounds since I last did this climb and it was time to reset the benchmark, provided I make it to the top, of course.

I did make it but not without a few breaks along the way. I had picked an extremely hot day to attempt this climb

(92F/33C). Foolish to the extreme! But if you know me at all . . . as I climbed the hill the temperature continued to rise, and by the time I had reached the peak I was exhausted and slightly dehydrated. And I still had to descend. I knew I had pushed this beyond where I should have and I knew caution was paramount on the descent. I was light headed and unsure of my footing. Another intelligent decision on my part! But, I did make it down, and I eventually made it back to the garden where I had left my friends to enjoy their afternoon. I hung my head for at least 30 minutes before I dared to attempt to drive. Nausea was a friend I didn't need but one that I'd acquired, like it or not. But soon, I was back in body as well as spirit, and I was able to savour the victory of the moment.

So we made our way back to Grande Prairie where we had a light dinner to complete our journey. The night for me was far from finished, as I enjoyed the company of a very good friend, and stimulating conversation that fed me better than any food could ever do. Food for the mind and food for the soul. The body had taken on as much as it could handle on this day. What a day!

Day 3. I stayed the same once again. I guess I was expecting my big day yesterday to show itself in the numbers but that was not the case. I'm feeling incredibly lethargic right now so I need to be careful. Up on the mountain one day and down in the valley the next. Not good. I need to level out real soon.

But of course I had to have breakfast at you know where, which was fine but I could tell this was going to be a trying day. I was feeling anxious and that is usually not a good sign.

I had a club house and garden salad for lunch and followed that up later with another visit to McD's for a McDouble, small fries, and Diet Coke. I've got to head home where it's safe before I blow this day entirely. I made it home but I gave in once more and ate a peanut butter sandwich at 10 pm that night.

So enough is enough! I headed over to Costco and picked up a bag of chicken breasts, and a bag of mixed veggies. Starting tomorrow, dinner will be eaten at home. At least that's the plan!

I have some big goals that I fully intend to meet. To do that I've got to get my focus back. Where I'm heading eventually, I'm going to need to be as healthy as I can be physically, mentally, and spiritually. And that's the truth!

Day 4. Stayed the same again. I'm not complaining though since I seem to have stabilized despite my screw ups. The first

20 pounds vacated once they realized they were no longer welcome. But, baggage still remains, and I have full intentions of throwing it out with the rest of the trash.

I believe I served notice to myself the other day when I made the long, hard trek to the top of Dunvegan. It was not without a degree of pain, but well worth it, as the pain of staying where I'm at right now is far greater.

I can't be driving to Dunvegan to conquer hills every day so it's time to embrace Muskoseepi Park once again. I used to run these trails daily and I need to find the jam to do it once again. Everything I need is here, whether it be short walks, long jogs, or stairs. I just need to do it!

In days past I used the Nordic ski trails as my backdrop, or O'Brien Park, or the Emerson Trail, and of course the Park to set up my runs. I didn't care how far it was, I knew I could make it. Confidence was at an all time high and now, well, it's not.

I did the usual breakfast thing and then I headed to the office. Work is rather slow for me at the moment but in this business it is par for the course. And that's not good enough. If I want to head south I have to produce so it's time I dig a little deeper.

And no sooner do I write the above words than the phone rings and I'm back in business. What a life!

Wendy's would provide lunch on this day, in the form of a bowl of Chili and cheese. I decided to give myself a break from dinner this evening but I did give in to a large soft ice cream and a handful of cherries.

Day 5. I'm still not losing any weight but I'm feeling great. It's time to see another loss on the scales so I'm being pretty diligent right now. I need results and I'm determined to get them.

I have a busy day in front of me but first I need breakfast. McD's was waiting for me with a McGriddle and a large Diet Coke to kick off my day. I have solemnly pledged to myself to eat only when I'm actually hungry, not just because it's lunch or dinner time. We will see.

Ok, I'm hungry. A McDouble, small fries, and pop took away the hunger pangs (if I even know what hunger pangs are), and I was back fighting the good fight.

I grabbed a power bar and a handful of cherries and I hit the road. I ended up in Eaglesham, strangely enough, at dinner time and of course I couldn't refuse their hospitality. So I did my best to force down the roasted chicken, rice, peas, and carrots. Oh, and I had to have some desert since I didn't want to insult my hosts!

Day 6. No McD's this morning but I did have breakfast with some friends. The problem with being out of my comfort zone, known as McD's, is that I always eat more than I should. I mean, how could I resist the 2 over easy eggs, the bacon, and the bagels topped with peanut butter and jam? I couldn't and I didn't.

I knew it was going to be a busy day. We were moving Mom to the Villa today so there was lots to do. And it was hot! Several hours later would find us at the local hotel chowing down. And of course, weak as I am, I gave in and ate a huge cheeseburger accompanied by fries with gravy, and Diet Coke. I have such good intentions but my flesh is weak!

A couple more hours of work and it was time to head back to GP. I fuelled up, and then on impulse, I grabbed a chocolate bar along with a Diet Coke to make the trip back home.

At last I'm at home writing this. To say that I'm unimpressed with myself is an understatement. One thing that has become abundantly clear to me while I'm on this self-imposed program is this: I need to stay in my own sandbox while I'm doing this. I stray far too easily!

Day 7. July 13. I gained back 2 pounds! I can't say I didn't deserve it. With only 4 days left in this 10 day challenge, I've got a lot of catching up to do. Of course, I'm at McD's writing this while consuming both a McGriddle and an Egg McMuffin along with a couple of Diet Coke. I might be down but I'm not out.

After church I stopped at McD's once again for a bran muffin and a pop. My intention was to head to the trails but it was way too hot so I decided to meet a friend instead. We decided to take in a movie which was fine, but once again, I loaded up with popcorn and pop. I justified it by making it my dinner. Good excuse, and then I headed home.

FLASHBACK

I've been involved in a long distance relationship for over 3 years now. I didn't think I was capable of such a thing, and yet here I am, totally committed to seeing this through. I've thought long and hard about this and why this is so different than anything that has went before. I've certainly been involved before, and married too many times, and I might add, judged accordingly, and yet this is different. In fact, everything about this is different.

She was incredibly beautiful but I chose to ignore that. And she was intelligent. Add in feisty and temptation quickly overtook common sense. I thank God everyday for bringing us together because this was, and still is, a relationship that should never have happened. There are many among us, on both sides of the equation, that would dearly love for this "thing" to fade away. We aren't among them. Our relationship grows stronger by the day, despite the obstacles. Whenever doubt rises it's ugly head, I need only look up to understand why this incredible relationship exists.

Day 8. The number on the scales is certainly indicative of the effort I've put in this last week. But, I guess it's not all about a "number," is it? I'm feeling good, a lot is being accomplished in all areas of my life, and I know with each passing day I am that much closer to being with Malena on a permanent basis.

As usual, I'm at my favourite haunt having my favourite breakfast, a McGriddle and a Diet Coke. Say what you will, it is my port in the storm, and as long as I'm in GP, it will remain thus. I added a parfait for good measure, I mean, I do like to eat healthy!

I had lunch with some friends today in the great outdoors, but once again, I was able to display my great will power and limit my intake to one delicious salmon sandwich topped off with 2 slices of cheddar, a couple of pickles, and a glass of iced tea. I do enjoy eating!

I AM A TRANSIENT

I've got to find a place to live yet again. If I was in a better position to just leave, to board that bird and fly away, that's what I would do. But I can't. At times like this, I'm disgusted with myself, I try so hard not to "go there" but I can't help wonder why this whole transition is taking so long if it's so important to me. Why aren't I accomplishing more? I am perplexed to my very core by my seeming inability to move beyond the status quo. And even as I write this, I know better. There is purpose in this life and I have mine, and like it or not, I am probably exactly where I'm supposed to be at this particular time in my life. Trust me, I am well aware of all the blessings that I have in my life, particularly all the incredible relationships. I could ask for nothing more in this area, and yet, I am sad. Very sad and very lonely.

And though I wax poetic, the fact remains, I need a place to live and I need it soon. I guess I'd better start taking this seriously. I wonder who would want me as a tenant? I'm here today and perhaps gone tomorrow. I don't want anything too comfortable or I may drag my heels even longer than I already am. I don't want to pay very much for rent as I require very little and because I'm trying to build up my escape fund. I'm certainly someone a landlord can count on, aren't I? This should be fun!

God I hate handcuffs! The irony is that no one even knows I have them on, and yet they bind me more securely than those of the visible variety ever could. To add further insult to injury, I hold the key, yet apparently I don't think I'm worthy of being free, at least not yet. How idiotic is that? If that was you telling me this, I'd have some choice words for you, starting with "Get over yourself!"

Perhaps I'd better reread the above paragraph a few dozen times. In any case, I went to CR this evening, and when it was over, I met my daughter for a walk around the reservoir and a date with the dreaded stairs. She was intrigued by my fascination with this seemingly innocuous appendage. But, after several trips up and down the staircase, she became a believer in the power of stair climbing to give one a workout like no other!

I just hope I follow my own advice and hit those suckers hard every other day. Knowing me, I probably won't.

Day 9. I think I'm back in the swing of things again. When I do the work, I get the results. Pretty simple formula, don't you think? I have some catching up to do but my mind is saying yes. We will see.

I'm writing this from McD's once again where I just consumed the best McGriddle ever. I'm still hungry but I'm heading to the trails for a bit. Those stairs are waiting for me so I best go. They beckoned me come, and come I did until I was exhausted! What a great feeling. And then I headed back to McD's for a breakfast burrito and a couple of glasses of water. Yes, water!

I'm feeling great at the moment. I'm busy with work; I've bought into this exercise program; my Moms' move was successful; my daughter has grown in leaps and bounds this last while, and my my eyes are fixed firmly on the goals I've set for myself here and abroad. It's an exciting time and this stone refuses to gather any moss. As if that wasn't enough, Malena just called to tell me how excited she was to get a load of topsoil for the yard! I mean, how does one top that!

When lunch rolled around I picked up a couple of bananas and headed to Crystal Lake. As usual, this became about a lot more than eating. On the dock stood a young lady that was obviously on a mission. She had rescued a gosling from a sure death in an oil pit at her work site and she was attempting to set the little guy free, hoping a mama duck would adopt him. But, she had to get back to work so I volunteered to do what I could while I was there. She gave me her number in the faint hope that I might have something positive to report to her. Well, I did. The little guy emerged in the open water so I captured a photo of him and sent it to her. I think that made her day and I believe she may have saved it's life.

I ate my bananas and then headed to McD's for a McDouble, fries, and pop before taking in an afternoon movie (the latest Transformers movie . . . how boring). What a waste of time!

Day 10. I'm down some more but I'll save the numbers for the official weight in tomorrow. And now I'm off to my haunt before heading to work for a bit.

After work I decided to hit the trails once again. 45 minutes later I'm drenched with sweat and it feels, oh so good. I know I'm making progress!

Went for a late lunch at McD's where I was joined by Christianah, a young lady from Nigeria who is over here studying to be a nurse. She tells me that I have to come to her wedding in Nigeria. I'm not so sure about that.

I headed back up to Crystal Lake to do some writing. I'm very focused right now on meeting my weight goal as well as completing my manuscript. And then the call comes. "The meeting is about to start." Oops!

After the meeting I headed off to spend some time with a friend before heading home for the evening. I'm hungry but determined not to blow all the work I've been doing this week on some impulse eating. If I was hungry that would be a different thing. I did compromise a little; I had a couple of tablespoons of peanut butter.

THE VERDICT

Well, I'm down to 248 pounds. I only lost 3.8 pounds over the last ten days but at least I'm back on track. After all, I'm down a total of 24 pounds since May 28th and my BP is currently 133/83.

THE SECOND TEN DAYS - STAGE 2

Day 1. 248 pounds. BP 133/83. It's cool today and it's early morning but I'm still heading to McD's. I'm really hungry today and, as is my habit, I seem to screw up the first few days every time I begin the next segment. Hopefully not this time. I say that, but I still added an extra McGriddle to the menu this morning.

I know I have my work cut out for me from here on in. I've lost nearly a half a pound daily since I began this ordeal and the weight will begin to come off even slower I'm afraid. I need to keep my focus.

I need to change the subject for a bit right now. I have incredible friends that accept me just the way I am, as I do them. As a result, we have some fascinating discussions about a lot of things, and they are never boring! We are all in such different places, and yet, we have a bond that is unlikely to be broken.

We come from different worlds, different cultures, different faiths, and yet we share common experiences which serve to bond us tightly together. We often wonder aloud what our lives may have become if we were more conformist. I think we agree that life would have been "easier" but we quickly dispelled that notice as we felt the "price" would have been too great. I love these kind of people!

And finally, after much persuasion, a very good friend of mine is taking the plunge and giving into that temptress called IPAD! She's a writer and I've been trying hard to convince her to give up the notebooks and give the IPAD a try. Well, she is! And I'm betting she will soon become very possessive of that device!

So today I wait. Another removal,of conditions is imminent. Piecemeal work can be frustrating but incredibly rewarding as well. I've made a choice to live in a world of peaks and valleys; it's incredibly edifying and I have a sense of freedom that knows few bounds provided that I do my part. On occasion, I haven't, and the self imposed handcuffs nearly cut off my circulation. Fortunately, I've been able rise up again and again and hold onto that dream of tomorrow that is edging ever closer to today.

I had some disturbing news from down south that added to my frustration at the slow progress that we seem to be making towards leaving this land of ice and snow. Yet, we hold on, for we know our hearts desire, and we will not be denied.

When I get agitated my natural tendency is to eat. So I'm at McD's again having a McDouble, small fries, and Diet Coke. I'm actually hungry so I'll cut myself some slack, in fact, I'm having a soft ice cream as well. So I'm emotional from time to time! Who isn't? Around 9 pm I gave in and had a handful of unsalted cashews and almonds, and then followed that up with a thick peanut butter sandwich. Darn!

I guess I'd better start thinking about a place to live while I'm here. I wasn't expecting to have to move again, but I do. That sucks but it's not my choice. If I was in a slightly different position I would get on that big bird and fly away. But, I can't. Not yet.

Day 2. Staying the same but that's ok. Back to McD's for my usual breakfast. It might seem like I'm thumbing my nose at convention but I'm not. I am deadly serious about losing the weight but I'm equally convinced that I don't have to have a steady diet of lettuce to achieve the results I want.

I'm hungry again! I've got to be so careful when I get this way. What to eat? Where? I guess the "where" is obvious, and no, I didn't have lettuce! I had a Sweet Chili McWrap, and for the record, it contains 410 calories, and 13% fat, and it was delicious!

Today should bring me a removal of conditions that is long overdue. And now, I've got to find a place to live!

I'm not in the greatest mood at the moment. In fact, I'm peed off at something I can do nothing about. That's probably a good thing as it would lead to a confrontation that would not end well. Enough said!

The last thing I wanted to do was to injure myself in any way that could possibly affect my weight loss journey. So wouldn't you know it? Last night I ran thigh on into a rather stationary device. Long story short, I am in major pain and I'm angry at myself for doing something so stupid! I assure you, this was not on purpose but of course there are consequences to every action, and I'll need to be careful that I don't use this as an excuse to "take it easy" and not do the things necessary to reach my goals!

Conditions were removed earlier today which makes me a very happy boy! It seems like it always has to be the eleventh hour in this business. The amount of work that goes on behind the scenes is monumental compared to what the client sees up front. I often liken it to a glacier. It's impressive and yet the bulk of it is hidden beneath the surface!

It's getting late but I'm not ready to go home yet. Well, actually I am, but alas, my home is far, far away. 6,000 miles to be exact, and that sucks! So instead, McD's will have to do. It's my sanctuary for the time being, plus I'm hungry, as usual. It's great to have a "safe house," office, meeting place, writing place, at my disposal most hours of any given day. Some of you understand this; most of you probably don't. I'm often asked how I could write in such an environment but the truth is, it seems to energize me. And besides, this place is an incredible microcosm of humanity brought together in one place for a finite amount of time. It's you; it's me, and that's exciting!

Day 3. Gotta love it! I'm down a couple of more pounds plus my blood pressure is 135/84. Life's good. I'm meeting some friends from McLennnan in a few minutes at Smitty's, but of course, I'm at McD's at the moment writing this. Can you imagine, they don't like McD's! What's with that? And since I've already eaten my usual gourmet breakfast here, I'll talk while they eat. Sounds like a pretty good deal to me!

The pain in my left thigh is excruciating. I'm sure it's bruised right down to the bone. It's ironic as I'm always so careful about where I place my feet or how I use my body to ensure that I don't hurt myself inadvertently. The last thing I need, particularly when I'm on this program is anything that could possibly interfere with me accomplishing my weight loss goals. Even though I'm not exercising a lot, at least I was constantly in motion, and this is screwing me up big time! But, I'll keep moving anyway, accompanied by pain as my walking partner. I don't really buy into the "no pain, no gain" mentality, but it's here now so I'll suck it up and see it through regardless.

I just had a great visit with another friend at McD's. Believe it or not, I didn't eat because I had designs on cooking myself a simple meal of grilled chicken breast and some mixed veggies. And that's what I did and it was excellent! I'm not much of a cook but I have to tell you, I did good! A handful of unsalted mixed nuts worked as desert. A good day overall.

Day 4. The weight continues to drop so I know that I'm in the zone. I wish I would notch up the exercise quotient a bit but I guess I really can't complain. The leg pain is really hard to take and walking is even proving difficult. I will not let this deter me though; I've come too far to let anything stop me. Naturally, I'm at "my place" sharing these thoughts and trying not to let this set back trigger any emotional eating. That's what usually kills me!

Many of the people I know wonder aloud why I'm still here. "Why aren't you in Panama with Malena?" I ask myself that question as well from time to time. It seems to be taking a very long time. I say that I'm fully committed to us and yet, here I am, and there she is. For a guy that is known for taking risks, I seem to be afraid to take the plunge. I don't believe there's anyone I know that doesn't think I'll do well wherever I go, and even I think that, but still . . .

I've thought long and hard about why I haven't left yet and I believe my reasons are sound. I have several things that need to be cleared up here or I'll be leaving unfinished business, and that is not wise. I also believe that the self induced program that I'm on can best be achieved here. I cannot discount the fact that timing is critical, and that patience is indeed a virtue, and that endurance will be vital to our ongoing success. I have tried mightily to surrender my will to Someone far greater than me, and trust the results. I believe that is happening. If it were not so, I don't believe I'd feel as contented as I now do. So, I am at peace as much as my humanity will allow. And of course, being me, tomorrow may find me in an entirely different space!

But, it's off to church. I'm definitely not religious but I am wholeheartedly a Christian. I love the sermons and they help keep everything in perspective. And then it's off to spend time with a friend. We always have interesting conversations and I doubt that this one will be any different.

And now I write, at McD's. I'm in a good space right now. Heck, I think I'll have a soft ice cream!

I decided that I may as well go home and dig out the George Foreman grill. I must say, with the addition of a little olive oil, and a few herbs and spices to punch up the taste, the grilled chicken breast was a winner! I added some broccoli, and cauliflower, and a few other assorted veggies, and all was good in my world! It's probably best I don't let too many people I know that I actually can cook or I'll get invited out less often. And besides, we wouldn't want McD's to go out of business, would we now?

So this lonely boy will have a couple of visits with different friends this evening. I really enjoy these visits, and I accommodate as much as I can because one day I will fly away to another part of the world and then these visits will have to take place electronically. I will always strive to keep in touch with those who want to be part of my life. Anyone who knows me well, knows this. As far as I'm concerned there is no good excuse not to keep in touch with others. If you don't, it's because you don't want to, or it's just not a priority. In that case, let's not waste each other's time.

Day 5. I'm down again (weight) and feeling good! Now for a couple of hours work. Im feeling so good that I think I'll take a road trip. And I did, and I ended up at Spring Lake at some fine friends where I'll stay the night.

But, before I leave GP, I need to head to McD's this morning for breakfast, and I did, and I ate way too much. It took 2 Bacon and Egg McGriddles to satisfy the craving, accompanied of course, by Diet Coke.

Travelling does make one hungry so we headed into Stony Plain to the local Boston Pizza. I have to tell you, that even though I wasn't in my own sandbox, I did good. A lemon salmon filet with a healthy side of veggies along with a salad bathed in a raspberry vinaigrette fit the bill perfectly! But of course we needed some desert so we headed over to McD's for a soft ice cream. It was so, so good!

We headed back to their acreage and spent the evening in the hot tub accompanied by some cold beer and great conversation. So it was late to bed, and early to rise. What a great day!

Day 6. Up at 6 am; McD's at 7. A few minutes later and I'd consumed 2 Egg McMuffins and a couple of Diet Coke. Then Ken headed to Edmonton and I took off for points west, first stop, Falher to see how my Mom was faring in her new place (she's doing great), and then a quick visit with Bruce before he headed to the dentist. And now I'm off to Watino for another quick visit with my sister and brother in law. I definitely don't outwear my welcomes this way! Their home is slated for demolition in the days ahead, the house I grew up in . . . and then I realized that I've never really grown up. I'm so confused!

And then another quick stop in Eaglesham and finally I was off to GP where an offer was waiting for me. I'm back in GP and my first stop has to be . . . you guessed it! The McDouble, fries, and Diet Coke found their place on my plate once again, and all was right with the world.

We managed to get an accepted offer and now both seller and buyer can move on with their lives. So now I write, and of course, it's at my favorited haunt.

Day 7. Staying the same but I'm not complaining. I strayed from my sandbox for a couple of days, and although I didn't lose any weight, I didn't gain any either. I call that a win!

In any case, it's time to get back on the horse. My leg is feeling quite a bit better so I'm hoping I can get back on the trails within a couple of days.

I thought I'd try and scale back a bit on my eating so I'm doubling up the eggs on the McMuffin and treating it like an open Denver to pretend that I'm actually having 2 of them. Sounds goofy but oh well! Of course I had to have a couple of Diet Coke. That's a non-negotiable.

2 pounds from now (30 pounds) will find me switching to a smaller sized drink. 12 pounds from now will see me switching to water instead of pop, at least that's the plan.

So I decided to throw in the shorts and the teeshirt, as well as the runners and head to the park. I was darn near there when the call came. "Can we meet you at the office?" I knew what they meant. "Can we meet you at McD's?" Of course. And that led to setting up an appointment with a Mortgage Broker. After introductions were made, I headed to the park, finally. So here I am, writing this, and polishing off a fruit and nut protein bar along with a healthy supply of water. It's a hot day but I'm liking it. I texted a friend my location but whether they join me or not remains to be seen.

I've got to get some papers signed up later today and I have another meeting slated for 5 pm today. And then I'll eat and NOT pig out!

I didn't! I had a Sweet Chili Wrap and a Diet Coke, but I admit, I did finish off a chicken breast that I had left over from the night before. A good, good day.

Once again I must reiterate, I am incredibly blessed to have so many wonderful friends in my life. I find it hard to understand when people speak of having very few, or no friends. I don't profess to know a lot, but I do know a little about this subject. When you are with someone, be fully engaged. Make them feel like they are the most important person in your life at that moment, because they are. You are sharing time together, and time is finite. Make your time significant. And, don't make it all about you. Remember, 2 ears, one mouth. Use accordingly. If you do this, I guarantee you will have more friends than you have time for.

I'm certainly finding myself in an interesting place these days. I need to move but I'm doing absolutely nothing about it. It's like pretending it doesn't exist so therefore it doesn't, but of course, it does. I want to move alright, but this is definitely un-expected. Frankly, it sucks! If I had a bit more jam, I'd say the hell with it and jump on a plane going to you know where! But, I've dug a bit of a ditch for myself and if I'm not careful, the ditch could become a grave. Oh joy!

Day 8. Down again. It's raining and I love it. Time to grab the camera and go for a drive to see what's waiting to be discov-ered by my camera and me. It's a constant reminder to myself to practice what I preach. Don't just look . . . learn how to SEE! And of course, I mean in all areas of my life.

But now it's time for breakfast and that can only mean one thing: McDonald's. A Bacon and Egg McMuffin with an extra egg added, plus my Diet Coke and all is right with the world. A long telephone conversation with Malena served as the dessert that would more than satisfy my cravings for the day.

I did find the scene I was looking for and my camera brought my vision to life before my very eyes. It's always there if I can take the focus off myself long enough to really see; to peer beyond the veil. Luck has little to do with it; seeing has everything to do with it.

Lunch found me back at my usual haunt as did a late din-ner. I know it seems ridiculous to anyone reading this that I could exist almost entirely on fast food, plus lose weight, but I assure you, everything I'm telling you is true. Every bite. I think I've got this figured out and yet I'm aware that these could be "famous last words" so I need to stay wary. The absolute key for me is portion control and no night eating.

This was another day with some amazing interactions that have become the "norm" for me. It's all about the "listening." If I listen to others and they know I'm actually interested, they'll tell their stories. And what stories they tell! Be interested in others, and be interesting yourself, and you will never be lonely. As someone who likes to talk, I've had to learn to respect the ratio of ears to mouth in all of us and use accordingly. Trust me, it works!

And now for a couple of scoops of peanut butter to finish off the evening.

Day 9. Once again an Egg McMuffin with an extra egg made its way down my gullet, accompanied by a breakfast burrito this morning. Once again, it's raining, but like I said before, I love the rain! So, my camera and I hit the road once again but with mixed results. I was just "off" a bit and as a result, I did get some photos but nothing spectacular. So it goes.

Of course, I had lunch, and then set about writing for a few hours. I can really get lost while I'm writing, almost the same as when I'm in pursuit of the "perfect" photo.

I'm looking forward to a visit with a great friend any time now. We've been through a lot together, and pretty much know how each other's minds work. Trials and tribulations have been many; we've commiserated when necessary and we've rejoiced when victorious. And, we've been able to converse about a subject near and dear to my heart that I can share with very few. It feels good to know that a few people have actually supported my vision from the very beginning. Trust me, there have been very, very few.

So we had a great visit, as usual, and once again, I'm alone. Almost always. Fortunately, I'm pretty good alone, but even so, I needed to have people around me. One of the ways that works well for me is to go to a movie. "Lucy" it was, and it was indeed strange, and a perfect distraction to finish off a most interesting day. Did I mention that I just had to have a buttered popcorn and a Diet Coke?

I decided to visit McD's one last time before heading home. Home. I wish I could go home. I can't. So, I'll sit here and write for a bit. Perhaps someone will want to chat. Or not. I want to write but I can't. This is beginning to suck, and then the phone rang. Malena. God how I miss her! But now I can go to my temporary home and dream the night away.

Day 10. I seem to be retaining a bit of fluid these days. I'm not eating to excess but the weight is not coming off either. I think I'd better pay a bit more attention to my eating, especially at night.

So I say, but I'm back at McD's this morning again chowing down on my usual. But soon I'm off to the park for a long walk with a good friend and then finally to the office. Gotta work if I ever want to get out of this country.

I wish I was busier but I'm not. I'm happy that my leg seems to be doing well but I have a tendency to push things a bit so I need to contain my boredom and stay away from the trails. Once a day is adequate for the time being.

Well that didn't last. I'm back on the trails but it's better than hanging around McD's and eating just for the sake of eating. I've done that many, many times, and it wouldn't be hard to do it again. I know me pretty well!

And once again the day comes to a close. Time to head home, which as you know, doesn't excite me one little bit, unless we're talking about my southern home, of course! Then I can get excited.

I have a bit of food that I need to use up at home anyway. Of course, that's the good food; the chicken breast, the veggies, the food I should be consuming daily. I think I'm just lazy. Yep, I think that's it.

Verdict: I gained back 4 pounds! And I deserved every one of them! I'm back to 254 pounds!

FLASHBACK

Malena and I knew that if we were to even have a chance at a life together, we would have to move to another part of Panama. That we did and David became our home base. I would be spending most of my time in Canada anyway, and David would offer her and the kids far better opportunities than Bocas.

We would set up our home and enrol the kids in good schools. Furthermore, we had better access to decent medical facilities and care. For the most part that has happened, but sickness seems to be ever present, and solutions seem to be evasive. Still, it's better than what they had, so we will count our blessings.

Malena has continued to build our home while I've continued to work in Canada. Our plans have certainly not worked out as well as I envisioned, but we continue to make the sacrifices required , knowing one day we will be together in our home. One day soon, we hope. Whether anyone likes it or not, and there are many who do not, this is our destiny. There is something far greater at work here than just the two of us, and we fully intend to bring our dreams to fruition.

THE THIRD TEN DAYS - STAGE 2

Day 1. I might as well be frank right off the bat. I'm not happy. I've been pretending that everything is going just peachy in the weight loss department but the truth is, it isn't. I'm not sure why, and I've analyzed the food intake over the last few days to see what has went awry, but I'm not sure anything has. What am I babbling about? I'm up four pounds! This has happened over the last two days, and as much as I tell myself to relax, it ain't that easy. The great fear for anyone on a diet is that they will wake up one morning and find themselves right back where they started, or worse. Ok, I haven't went over the edge yet, and I can assure you, I won't. But, it's extremely frustrating!

I know all about plateaus and so on, and that may be what this is, but I suspect that what it really is is fluid retention. The types of food I eat, though limited in quantity, are of the high sodium variety. So today, I will make a conscientious effort to do something about that.

Of course, I'm at McD's writing this and having my usual breakfast. I added in some grapefruit for good measure, after all, I am trying to eat healthier. Today I expect great things out of me and I need to get back on track. My leg is feeling pretty good and excuses have no place in my life anyway. If I can't do one thing, I can certainly do another. Sixty days have now passed and I'm in danger of not meeting my goals if I don't get my act together.

I must admit that I'm letting stress get the upper hand on me as I deal with finding a place to live as well as dealing with the economic pressures that don't seem to want to let up. I'm an incredibly positive guy normally, but this is getting to me big time. Suddenly Panama seems a great distance away. It's supposed to be getting closer but it's not working out that way.

I do know how much I've been blessed in this life and I try not to ever forget it, but I do. I'm quite human, you know! I say I've surrendered, but in truth, not nearly as much as I need to. I know I'm all over the place as I'm writing this, but I need to get this down before I lose my thoughts. I am definitely on a voyage of self discovery, and have been since my conception. I'm quite convinced of that! The longer I live, the more I discover about myself and my motives, and fortunately, I can say that I do like me better today than I did yesterday. But putting feelings on paper is still a tad uncomfortable and I'm never sure how far I should take this. Being vulnerable is not a comfortable place! Not at all!

The church service was great again today, particularly when it ends with several baptisms. It's exciting to see people making a public declaration of their faith. Talking the talk is one thing; walking the walk, quite another. Now, if they can just avoid becoming religious . . .

So it's off to McD's for a double cheeseburger and a couple of large Diet Coke and a bit of writing. And then I'll hit the trails. I know that this funk I'm in won't go away on its own. It's time to get those endorphins firing and I know exactly how to do that! Plus, I may have found a place to live! I should know for sure this afternoon. When I force myself to surrender and quit trying to force issues, good things happen. I don't know why I have to go through this exercise every single time. You'd think I'd get it but obviously I'm a slow learner!

So I head home to change into shorts and a tee shirt and then I hit the trails. And then the call comes " Can you meet us for lunch at TR's?" You bet.

I'm offered a place to live until I take my leave to head down south. What a relief! Plus, there are no strings attached. When I just slow down and let patience guide me, the results are so much better. The couple that just extended the offer know me pretty well, and took it upon themselves to meet a need they knew I was struggling with. Thank you so very, very much.

I'm very sensitive about intruding on other people's space. I never take anything for granted and I don't assume a whole lot. I'd much rather leave early and be welcomed back than overstay my welcome in any and all circumstances. If I make an error, I want to err on the side of caution. And that's just the way I am.

And now I'm off to the trails. It's not a great workout but at least I know my mind is in the right place and when it is, my body will follow. It did, and I feel great! Ok, my leg is pretty sore but I can feel myself getting stronger. Onward and upward from here on in!

Finally dinner. A bowl of Chili followed up by a banana and a protein bar took care of today's culinary needs. I think today is a turning point once again, and now I'm heading straight ahead to the goal line!

Day 2. Well, I'm doing terrible! If I don't get my act together soon I'm in real danger of screwing this up completely. But of course, I'm writing this from McD's where I just had an Egg McMuffin with an extra egg, and get this, a banana, and of course my Diet Coke.

And now I'm off to Watino to watch the home I spent much of my youth in being demolished. It's best before date has long since passed, I'm afraid. Soon a new structure will occupy it's place and that's just the way it is. It was my parents home, but it came time for them to move into a seniors residence, and consequently, my sister and brother in law purchased and moved into the old abode. That was a number of years ago, and a decision had to be made. They made theirs, and as a result, here we are today.

There are some mixed emotions around this day, I'm sure. Dad has since moved on to his permanent home, and Mom continues to reside in the home they retired to. I know she certainly has some strong feelings about the homes demise, but she plays everything close to her chest. My sisters are constantly trying to figure out what "Mom really thinks about this or that." Like I said, she doesn't reveal a lot. Guaranteed, she won't be here to witness the destruction of her longtime home, that much I know!

But while I was there, my sister decided to grill some burgers. She's a great cook, so I was obligated (of course), to eat 3 burgers and 2 helpings of potato salad. Oh boy! But, I didn't want to hurt her feelings, after all! You know, as soon as I leave my own sand box, I'm in trouble. And since I'm in trouble anyway, I might as well pick up a chocolate bar and a muffin to eat on the way back to GP.

But nonetheless, it was a special day. it's Malena's birthday today, and even though we are far apart, we are closer together than most people could possibly understand. Again, it is what it is. And by the way, I didn't eat anything else today!

Day 3. If I thought I was doing terrible before, well, now it's even worse. This book project is going to turn into a joke if I don't get this figured out real soon! Of course, I'm writing this while enjoying a Bacon, Egg, and Cheese McMuffin and a couple of large Diet Coke. So what! I still have to eat, don't I?

It promises to be a busy day today and that is always good. If, or when I get a chance, I'm heading to the trails. And then the call comes. We need you to book a stress test. What? So I did for later this afternoon. Weird. I've been up to the top of Dunvegan. I've been hitting the trails regularly and I've felt great doing it. Plus, I've lost a pile of weight. I can't wait to see what this is all about.

A friend called to meet me for lunch at TR's. But I did good, real good. The Asian salad with the grilled chicken was perfect! See, I do eat salad on occasion!

"Ok Doctor, what's up?" "We need to run some tests on your heart." Excuse me. "I'm sorry, but something is not quite right. We're concerned." Ok, but I'm not sharing this info with any-body, at least not yet. Even then, I doubt that I'll share much. People get strange around you when they think there's some-thing wrong, or they want to treat the person like they're an in-valid. Sorry, wrong guy! I have a life and I fully intend on living it!

Still, it is disconcerting to say the least. And of course, I have no choice, do I? To go for the tests. If you know me at all, you'll know where I'm going with this. Perhaps it's best if I just drop the topic for now.

So I'll head back to McD's for a bit. As much as I try to push this aside, it's really bugging me. My God, we've worked so hard and made so many sacrifices already to even have a chance to be together, that the last thing we need is another mountain to climb! I'm starting to get angry and yet, I know that solves nothing, and besides, there may be nothing to be concerned about. Yeah, right! Oh well, time to have a McDouble, small fries, and Diet Coke, maybe 10 of them!

Day 4. I'm gaining weight, not losing it. Mentally, I'm extremely frustrated, and this latest news seems to have paralyzed me. I know I have to stay the course and I need to be careful who I speak to of this latest obstacle. So, I met a friend at the park this morning for a long chat. This is the kind of friend that I can really talk to, and talk we did. How often it seems that one step forward is quickly swallowed up by two steps backwards? When is enough, enough? I do understand the power of patience, and I do understand the necessity of endurance. And, I understand the power behind surrendering, and I understand just getting on with it . . . despite the circumstances but I also understand that I'm getting tired. Really tired.

In any case, I took a short road trip with another friend and ended up at Joey's Only for a couple of pieces of fish and chips. Interestingly, this particular friend, made a comment to me that I never really open up, that I keep everyone at a safe distance. I'm not sure how true that is, and I certainly open up more to some than others, usually with very good reason. I don't see anything wrong with that! I mean, it all depends on the subject, the degree of our friendship, and even my sense of how you will react in a given situation. If you're the type to over react, gossip, or are a know it all; if you're the type of friend that says you're there for me, but then you're not (unless it fits into your schedule), then don't expect much from me. Just be glad that I don't treat you the way you treat others. Enough said!

Well, the Doctor's office called and they already have me booked for tomorrow morning at 8:45 for an echocardiogram. No fooling around with these people!

But, the day isn't done yet. Another call came and another friend just asked me to come over to his place for dinner. How can I refuse? Of course, I don't. It seems like I'm always eating but really, I'm not. And I never, well, hardly ever, eat at night and I can't remember the last time I had chips or cheezies, and for me, that's a big deal!

Day 5. My diet is an absolute disaster! I've gained back several pounds this last week. I'm not even sure what to blame it on, as if that would make any difference anyway! In any case, I'm off to see my Doctor which should reveal a bit more about whether I have something to be concerned about or not.

The appointment went well and now I await results. Within the hour another call comes informing me of the date and time of the aforementioned stress test (August 18 @ 10 am). This whole thing is strange. I think I'll wait until I know more before I even mention this to Malena or my family. For now, I'll share with a few friends that may not panic as much.

But it's off for breakfast now and then it was time to head to the office. I'm awaiting a removal of conditions, which can be quite frustrating, since there's absolutely nothing I can do but wait for it. I hate that part. Too bad, so sad. Patience, my friend, patience!

I decided to head to the park with a bag lunch during the dinner hour today. A call from Malena brightened up a slightly overcast sky, that is, until she told me that she was on the way to the hospital with her son. They have so many medical issues between them that I refuse to have her worry about mine as well. I'll tell her later once I've had time to digest whatever they tell me.

A long day of waiting. The removal may come tomorrow. For now, there's nothing else that can be done. Patience required.

I finally decide that it's time to change and head down to the park. I'm pretty good at finding excuses NOT to do anything. That's got to change if I want to even come remotely close to meeting my goals. But I did make it once around the trails. Good on me!

And finally, it's dinner time but I kept it to a minimum. A Grilled Chicken Snack Wrap, Diet Coke, and a soft ice cream would be my meal. Maybe this day will be a new beginning once again.

And then I made one final trip to the trails to hit the 29 Steps of Hell to test out the leg. I made it up and down 10 times before calling it a day. That was intense but oh, so satisfying! Yes!

I made the mistake of sharing this little tidbit of info with a good friend this evening. Turns out that that was unwise. Let me summarize: "Are you a complete idiot? A little denial perhaps?" A slight pause, and then "Correction: a lot of denial." Ok. I got it. But this I know: I will not live in a state of fear. I can't, and I won't do it!

It's 9 pm and I'm still writing at you know where. I'm meeting another friend for a chat before I call it a day. Time to head home, wherever that is. I am truly a transient!

Day 6. I think it's going to be a good day. I'm still up a few pounds from my lowest a week ago but it's starting to come down again. I think stress has been rearing its ugly head a wee bit. Not sure about that, and I haven't been eating as well as previously, but at least I stayed completely away from junk food (my definition).

McD's is not junk food in my estimation so I'm eating my usual breakfast before I head out for a walk with a friend. And then it's off to work to once again begin the long wait for the removal of conditions that has to be removed today. Please!

The wait is excruciating but I seem to have enough friends that keep trying to distract me while I consume some McD's food over lunch.

And now it's 4 pm and I'm still waiting. I don't like this one bit! And then the call comes: "We need an extension." Oh great, but at least the deal is still alive. And that's the way it goes in this business.

I had dinner with my daughters to finish off the day so that was great. It's nice to do something regular once in a while.

Except the day wasn't finished. I headed down to Muskoseepi Park where the 100th Anniversary of Grande Prairie celebrations were taking place. There is some incredible talent in this area and some of these people are my friends. It adds a special touch watching people you know perform before thousands of people.

But of course, they wanted to go eat. It's late and they're hungry. I went with them, and I know it's hard to believe, but all I had was WATER! It's true. I can do this!

Day 7. Since I was so good last night I knew I could now have the breakfast of champions this morning, which of course meant an Egg McMuffin with an extra egg and a copious amount of Diet Coke plus a breakfast burrito. I didn't lose any weight but I sure am feeling better!

I did a bunch of running around to complete the morning and then I met a friend for lunch. It must seem that all I do is eat. An Asian salad accompanied by a beer (horrors) definitely set up the rest of the day.

I finally made it to McD's this afternoon so I could do some serious writing. I schedule my writing the same as any other appointment because it keeps me on track. Perhaps one day you'll buy this book and when you come across this part, you'll know that my discipline actually paid off. I have to assume that if you've got this far into this book that you understand my journey, and it is probably not all that dissimilar from yours. Read on! Meanwhile, I'm going to have lunch!

It went downhill from there. Well, kind of. I went to the park again tonight until around 10 pm before heading home. I thought I had this night well in hand but I couldn't resist having a cheese sandwich and a handful of cashews before retiring. Darn! I'll probably pay. I know I can't eat at night. Ever!

Day 8. Of course, I paid. Big surprise. But I refuse to give up on McD's. It's certainly not their fault. I know exactly who is to blame. So I'm off to McD's for a quick breakfast and then off to a friend's church. I love different cultures and I love the fact that even though I'm white, I seem to fit in everywhere. I certainly hope that's true because I plan on coming back here a bunch more times. What rhythm they have; too bad I didn't!

And then I was off to spend time with a good friend before I headed back down to the park. I'm incredibly restless these days so I have to keep moving. The best way for me to do this is to be around others, and with all the activities going on at the park this weekend, it was a no brainer.

Time to eat. I heard McD's calling my name so I answered, as usual. But, I ate way too much. I really don't understand me!

I say I want to reach this goal in the worst way and yet I keep sabotaging myself.

I headed down to the park one last time to see the grande finale which culminated with a huge fireworks display. I guess the good part is that I spent a lot of time with friends this weekend. The sad part is that I want to spend a lot more time with Malena, and that is just not happening!

Day 9. It's been a great weekend and last nights fireworks were the icing on the cake. But then I jumped on the scales and the reality of my weekend slapped me in the face. I deserved nothing less! So I'm at my usual place writing this and deciding where to go from here. After all, Malena likes me just the way I am. Maybe I don't need all this bs! I know! I know! Crazy talk! Anyway, enough! I move tomorrow so I've got lots to do today. Onward.

It's really important that I stay active physically so I'll be hitting the trails in short order. Despite my setbacks, and there have been many, I will succeed. I really do believe that I can make a living writing but I need proof of that. I need to get these books out there and prove it to myself. Perhaps I'm procrastinating so I don't have to face the reality that I'm just not good enough. Who knows! And yet, if it were to work, I could live anywhere in the world and make my living. I'm great at encouraging others to go for it, but a bit of a procrastinator when it comes to myself. Perhaps I'm just a hypocrite. I tell others to let faith rule, not fear, and yet I'm doing exactly the opposite! What a guy!

I am soaking wet. From sweat if you can believe it! I did a pile of work around the yard and that my friends, definitely qualifies as a workout! That's two hard earned showers today so far and a third is on its way. Yes!

Man, is it hot! Trust me, I don't ever complain about the heat but this is intense. Nonetheless, I'm down at the park doing some writing. I've been really careful about my food consumption so far today but it's time for a protein bar and a gallon of water. When I'm good, I'm really good!

In any case, I'm off to a meeting shortly, and even though there will be lots of food there, I'm feeling good and back in control. Just to make sure that I don't fall off the wagon, I brought along another protein bar. Can't be too careful! I'm aware that most of this diet stuff is about mindset and I think I've reset mine.

I managed to make it home without further incident and I'm happy to call this day a success. Hopefully it's reflected on the scales as well!

Day 10. Finally! Things are starting to turn around! With only 10 days to go I've got to stay focused, and you know what, I will. Tomorrow morning I'll officially weigh in again, I'll re-group as I do every 10 days, and begin again.

I move today and that sucks but it is what it is. Thank God some great people stepped up and saved me from being a full blown transient (ok, I know that's being a wee bit dramatic). Seriously, I feel totally displaced. ET go home should read DD go home!

But with each passing day I get closer and closer to doing just that. We know exactly what we have to do, and we are doing everything we can to make our life a reality. The right attitude is paramount and so far, we have that in spades.

In any case, I'm at McD's once again polishing off my usual breakfast. A quick stop at the office is in order and then I'm off to pack and to make another move. I pray this is the last one before "the big move."

What a hot day! I'm not complaining, mind you, this is merely a precursor of what I will be living in on a daily basis in the near future.

At least I'm done moving. Kind of. My vehicle is packed, my bed is in pieces at the new place. I stink (I'm sweating like a porker), but I'm heading back to McD's for a couple of large, cold, Diet Coke. I find that if I'm on the ball I only eat enough to satisfy my hunger, not eat just for the sake of eating. That's exactly what I used to do, and my weight rose accordingly. Trust me, I'm still very capable of slipping into the abyss at any time.

I'm exhausted from the move, both mentally and physically, but I'm on track and feeling pretty darn good about it. I'm starting to get really excited and I can't wait to see some good results on the scales tomorrow morning!

It's weird going to another new place tonight. I'm getting really tired of this. I want to go home and I want to go now! But, for now, I'm exhausted and the bed looks oh so good. I'm so doggone sore that I may not be able to pry myself out of bed in the morning. But I will. I'm anxious to jump on those scales!

THE VERDICT

Well, I'm kinda happy. The scales say 242 pounds which works out to .43 pounds per day over 70 days. I wanted more but I certainly didn't deserve more. I have to take this more seriously!

THE FOURTH TEN DAYS - STAGE 2

Day 1. I'm feeling good and feeling bad all at the same time. I'm making progress but at a lot slower pace than I expected. Time is going by and I've got a long ways to go yet. Let's begin.

I switched to the medium pop today as I promised myself. Not that it'll make any difference. And yet, I probably shouldn't say that. After all, I switched from Big Macs to McDoubles and smaller burgers; I switched from large fries to small fries; I switched to breakfast McWraps from McGriddles; I cut out the hash browns and hot cakes for the most part, and I will often turn a McMuffin into an open Denver to trick myself just enough to keep my eating contained. I know that a lot of people will cringe at the above sentence but that's their problem, not mine.

Ok, I need to focus. I really want to head out on a road trip but I think I'll rein that in for a few more days. I'm much safer if

I stay in my own sandbox. With less than 20 days to go, I don't want to screw up now.

Malena and I chat daily, often just for a couple of minutes at a time, but it keeps us connected. We seem to have an incredibly strong bond that is serving us well. We have a lot of opposition but as long as we stay committed to each other the way we are, we will win this battle of wills.

We certainly find it frustrating at times. Progress is painfully slow. Without her attitude towards life, I doubt we could do this. I want to just go for it, dive in (and probably sink), but she is the solid one. She is so practical, the ying to my yang. I may be older but she is far more mature. I wonder what that says about me?

I'm certainly not blogging like I used to. It was a great release and it helped me focus on other things besides "poor me." I keep wanting to switch my blog towards my novel writing but I can't seem to figure out what the heck I'm trying to do. I guess if I ever figure it out I'll go for it. Or perhaps I'll start a new blog. Or not. I'm so confused!

Time for a walk with a few stairs chucked in for good measure. I'm so flipping tired yet from the move but I soldiered through anyway. I want this real bad!

And finally I'm home but it's way to early to go to bed. So I head out to the deck to write. If I went to bed now, I'd be up by 3 am. Forget that!

Day 2. I had a great sleep, and no, I didn't get up at 3 am. And now I'm ready to rock! So it's off to McD's so I can start this day off properly.

Sore or not, I'm heading down to the trails. Failure is not an option. Then Malena called and that always puts me in a happy place. Life is good. Well, kind of.

It just got better. The letter I was waiting for arrived. Yes! I'm going on a road trip after all.

Of course, I had to eat first, so I headed to, well, you know where. The Egg McMuffin with an extra egg, and the breakfast burrito hit the spot perfectly and I was off to points north.

I hit Falher in time to meet a friend for lunch but I was a good boy. A bowl of soup and a Diet Coke took care of my culinary needs just fine, thank you very much.

This was just a one day road trip and I was determined that it wouldn't screw up my diet. I took evasive action and instead of picking up some junk food to snack on on the trip back to GP, I headed to the Co-op and bought a head of red cabbage which I had them quarter, and that served as my snack on the way home. I also made a pit stop at my sister's place and raided her pea patch as well as borrowed a couple of kohlrabi to munch on. I am so health conscious!

I'm back in GP at McD's where I had to have a Diet Coke. After all, that's my addiction and I have to feed it! Sorry, it's true. And now it's time for a walk before I head home.

I'm home and I'm tired, but I'm feeling oh so good. Bed time at last . . . and then the phone rang. And off I went. But, I didn't eat another bite.

Day 3. Another 8 days to go and I'm getting excited. I'm doing well at the moment and I want this real bad. I'm my own worst enemy so I have to be really careful from here on in.

A regular day turned into a rather late night last night so I didn't get to McD's until 8:30 this morning. That's late for me but I'm rocking right now and sleep is the last thing on my mind.

I forgot that the office was closed today but in my line of work it doesn't really matter. I still removed conditions on a deal I was working on so I'm happy, and my clients are happy, and that makes for a very good day.

Time for lunch. I'm meeting Aaron at Tito's for some incredibly healthy food in the form of Chicken Souvlaki. It was absolutely delicious, and no, I'm not giving up on McD's. Not a chance!

My diet is going really well and I'm convinced I'm going to finish this race in fine fashion. I'm very aware that a diet is about a heck of a lot more than just food. My attitude needs to undergo a transformation as well so I'm hoping that that is taking place along with the weight loss.

With the weekend approaching it becomes tougher sticking to it, but I absolutely need to. I keep repeating this over and over but I need to: I want this real bad!

I'm in it to win it and I know the only thing that can sabotage it is ME! I can almost smell victory!

Day 4. It turned out that I wasn't finished with yesterday after all. Some friends called and invited me for dinner. I accepted graciously and helped myself to steak, potatoes, peppers, mushrooms, salad, and Saskatoon pie topped with ice cream. And a glass of wine. The food was great and the company, equally so. Thank you so much for the invitation!

I didn't weigh in this morning. I decided to give myself a break after the rather large dinner I consumed last night. It's funny how I begin to feel guilty about what I eat until I realize that I'm doing quite fine, thank you very much!

But that doesn't stop me from heading to McD's for breakfast once again. And then off to the park for a walk and chat with a great friend. As usual, a 15 minute walk turned into an hour discussion!

It was business as usual for the rest of the day, interrupted only by a short lunch break that I admit, contained a few items I usually avoid. The smoothie was fine, but the pizza and the hotdog? Questionable at best. Oh well, what's done is done.

The dinner hour was upon me and I was getting ready to screw up today's diet when the phone rang and a friend invited me to hit the trails with him. Yes! I have to admit, I didn't want to but I knew it was the cat's meow! It took my mind completely off the food and onto the walk and conversation that ensued.

I did make it back to McD's a bit later for another conversation and a couple of Diet Coke. But, no food. If I would have been really hungry I would have eaten, but I knew I was going to feed something besides my stomach and I wasn't about to let that happen. A victory of sorts.

In any case, it's time to head home. I did well today and I'm looking forward to the results tomorrow. And now there are only 6 days left on this stage.

Day 5. I met a couple of friends for breakfast this morning. I had my usual before heading to church. The service was held down in the park today, and after church, a BBQ would follow. Of course, I had to stay and eat. I certainly don't want to be rude!

And then I hit the trails for an hour or so. But I was still hungry and I knew this would be a trying day. I headed back to McD's where I managed to consume a bran muffin and 2 ice cream cones! Oh boy! I'd better stop right now or my goal will definitely be in jeopardy. There aren't a lot of days left so I can't be screwing up now! My mind is playing games with me big time!

It's way to early to head home yet. I need gas. I might as well grab a bag of cheezies. It can't hurt. I'm self sabotaging and I'm going to pay. And there's only 5 days left.

Day 6. I paid big time for my indiscretions over the past few days. I think I've dug a pretty big hole for myself. Suddenly my goal seems a long ways away and my chance of reaching it is remote. That sucks big time! Why do I do this to myself? I'm not giving up but I'm getting really discouraged.

On August 16th I'll weigh in and accept the results. What choice? I have a number in mind that I'm striving for, a realistic number I think, and I can still reach it but it'll require me to be absolutely perfect from here on in.

Of course, even though I write the above, I'm at McD's eating my usual breakfast. I want to reach my goal but I'm not above to starve myself! As if that would ever happen!

I'm off to the office. We're moving so it's time to purge. We're moving to a "virtual" office so there is absolutely no room for "stuff." Frankly, that sucks. By the same token, it's actually a good thing and helps ease me towards the door. When the time comes, it should be relatively easy to dump the remaining "stuff" and get on that bird and fly away to the land I want to call home.

I'm purging in all areas of my life, from the so called diet I'm on, to the personal possessions I own, to the absence of a "real" office and the embracing of my virtual life which I've been doing anyway, especially in the area of writing.

Once again, I'm dedicating myself to getting my diet back on track. There will be no more eating just for the sake of eating. No way! Of course, I'm making this vow from McD's where I just had a Grilled Chicken Snack Wrap and a couple of Diet Coke.

I hit the park earlier today with a friend for a long walk, and if I'm smart, I'll do that at least once more today. I need to walk more and eat less if I want to finish this self induced race with my head held high. It ain't over till it's over . . . and it ain't over yet!

I started checking flights again today. I know I probably shouldn't be doing that just yet but I'm really feeling lonely these days. I have lots of friends but I need to spend some time with Malena, and I have to do it soon. We will survive this drought like we have all the others, but it is too soon to move there permanently. I'm thinking next spring, possibly sooner, but I have to be careful not to set myself up for a big disappointment if it doesn't happen in my time frame. She is so much better at handling this than I am. I can't believe how much I learn from her. Even now, she throws out the caution "Duane, don't do anything foolish. You know what happened before." Of course, she's right. I've thrown caution to the wind on several occasions and ended up nearly being stranded in countries that weren't mine. Crazy indeed, but I like to think that the correct term is "good crazy."

Day 7. I'm down a few more pounds but I'm certainly not where I want to be. With only 4 days remaining in this stage the pressure is definitely on. Can I make my stated goal? It's unlikely. In any case, I'm at McD's writing this while I'm eating my usual breakfast. I'm extra hungry this morning so I'm overdoing it once again. I know I should be feeling bad about this but I don't. Seriously. I absolutely refuse to starve myself just to get the numbers to work even thought it's extremely tempting to do so.

I have a very busy day ahead of me, and given my current state of mind, that is a very good thing. I've also tossed in the shorts and tee shirt so I can hit the trails later. I've learned to eliminate all of my excuses of why I can't do something. If I don't follow through, it's because I didn't want to. Simple as that.

Time is flying by and I've got absolutely nothing done. Well, that's not quite true. I did hit the trails with a friend for a workout and an extended chat. My friends are so incredibly different one from another and I love it! It definitely keeps me sharp. Iron sharpens iron.

Another call and another meeting with a young chap who is on a self professed journey of discovery. It's an exciting thing to see and I do hope he keeps in touch. His last day in GP is on Friday and then he's off. I'm intrigued to see where his journey takes him!

I'm continuing the purge today, in all areas of my life, including my eating and exercise. Out with the crap and in with the good stuff. So sayeth I!

I'm meeting another friend at the Reach shortly but I'm not eating. I'll drink (pop), but I refuse to eat, unless I'm legitimately hungry. We will see.

This purging thing sucks! Either that, or I'm just really bad at it. And then another friend called and wants to go to the movies this evening. I'm in! But to make sure I don't screw up too badly I'm heading to McD's right now for a couple of Grilled Chicken McWraps. Better that than buttered popcorn at the movies. May the purge continue unabated!

Day 8. The movie was great (Guardians of the Galaxy) and I managed to stay away from the popcorn! In any case, I'm now down to the last 3 days of this stage, and even though I've plateaued and not likely to reach my goal, I can accept the results for what they are. How mature of me!

I got off to an early start today so of course I headed to McD's. I have to admit that I kind of overdid it a bit, so instead of 1 Egg McMuffin with an extra egg, I doubled up. I seem hell bent on self destruction right now. I know that what I ate would be fine as long as I stopped there. My history has shown that I'm all over the place with my eating. And yet I say that I'm committed to this goal and that the goal that I reach is really just the starting place for the next challenge that will follow the end of the first. There's a lot riding on this so I have to be careful not to downplay its significance.

The purging continues at the office. I should be done by day's end, except for the computer, a few files, and the telephone. My work space will be reduced to nothing more than a couple of file boxes. Something like the direction my personal life is going. Soon, there will be nothing holding me back, certainly not "stuff" and then I will prepare to go. My dream awaits me and it is not here.

Time to head back to the office for an hour or so and then I'm off to meet a friend for a long walk in the park. If I want to meet this goal I've got to spend as much time as I can in the park. When I'm there, I'm on; when I'm not, I slack off pretty quickly.

As usual, the chat was great, and though it seems I spend an inordinate amount of time with friends, I consider it to be a privilege spending time with those who wish to spend time with me. One day I will leave and the last thing I want to do is miss spending time with the significant people in my life. I believe nothing happens by chance in life and that people come into our lives exactly when they're supposed to. They may have a message for me; I may have a message for them; perhaps it goes both ways. In any case, I am always open to that possibility and do my best not to get so wrapped up in myself that I miss the opportunity to interact with others. I think I've missed many opportunities in the past and I will do my best to minimize those in the future. There is purpose in this life and I fully intend on living out mine.

It's time for dinner and McD's is once again calling my name. The Sweet Chili Wrap hit the spot, along with Diet Coke of course. Did you know that the wrap is not only low in calories and low in fat, but that it's also delicious! What else can I say?

I'm getting tired of spending so much time alone! I'm good at being alone but I crave companionship, especially Malena's, and she is so very far away! My patience is definitely wearing thin and I admit, I'm starting to get depressed. And that is not good when one is trying to lose weight!

So I write. I don't know what else to do with myself. It's too early to go home, wherever that is. I feel like I'm an alien dropped off at a planet that doesn't know what to do with me. Hell, I don't even know what to do with me. So I guess I'll just write.

But finally it's time to call it a day. I had a great chat with Patti when I got home, and then I got a call from Bob, my friend that I'd met in Costa Rica. Bob and his wife were with me when I first met Malena and can vouch that she actually exists. My kids have talked to "someone" on the phone whom they assume is her, and a couple of Canadian friends living in Panama have actually not only met her, but had invited us to dinner one afternoon. Of course, she ensured that they heard her side of the story, just to ensure that they were getting the real account of our story, you know, the true version. Imagine that! As if I would distort the truth! After dinner, when we were ready to depart, they gave us a gift. An appropriate gift, I might add. A machete. And now we have 2! Thank you very much!

It's time for bed. I did well today and I pray the results will manifest themselves on the scales tomorrow morning but I've learned to expect the unexpected. I guess we'll know in about 8 hours from now.

Day 9. And then there were 2 days left. I must admit, I'm relatively happy with my progress at the moment. But of course, I'm at McD's writing this again and chowing down on an Egg McMuffin and a breakfast burrito. I ain't giving these things up without a fight! Ok, I will when I get to Panama, but that's still a ways away.

I just heard some terrible news about a missing person who just happens to be the grand daughter of some dear friends of mine. The rumour mill is going crazy and the projected outcome is anything but positive.

I love my IPAD. It's fast, small, and does pretty much anything I need it to do. And right now, it's allowing me to work on a real estate course in the comforts of my favourite eating establishment. Thank God it's in modules so I can more or less do it on the fly. And I can eat an ice cream at the same time.

I moved a bunch more stuff today, and if I keep this up, I'll have it wrapped up in the next couple of days. And then I'll finally have enough room in my vehicle to store my bike. There goes another excuse that I've used from time to time NOT to get my butt in gear! There was a time where I refused to let excuses bog me down.

So I always ensure that I have an extra set of clothes in my vehicle, especially work out clothes, running shoes, and so on. And now my bike. I've fully committed myself to this lifestyle change, which actually is a reflection of what I would do routinely in the past.

I've been thinking about the changes I need to make in the near future, and I believe they are achievable. I fully intend to pick up the exercise quotient substantially; I intend on finally dumping the reliance on Diet Coke; I intend to improve my eating habits (eating at home a lot more; more fruits and veggies, etc.); and I intend on dropping a lot more weight. I know this is somewhat vague, but I will shore it up in the days to come.

In addition to the above goals, I will publish my book or be very close to having it ready to go in the next couple of months. I will also put in some serious effort into getting some of my photos published or at least get a working plan in place. Again, these appear vague but they will be firmed up in the days ahead.

But now I'm hungry and I want to hit the trails before I head home. A quick trip to McD's satisfied the cravings and the trails did the rest. And that's the kind of day it was.

Day 10. And here we are. The last day before the next official weigh in. I'm not doing as well as I hoped I would and yet I'm actually doing pretty darn good. It's really hard not to make this about a number but I'm trying to do just that. That's what I say but if the number falls short tomorrow, I know I'll be disappointed.

I was definitely overtired last night when I headed home, and as a result, I made a huge boner that could have been serious. I signalled, and when appropriate, I turned right into a one way street, going the wrong way! Oh oh! Vehicles were speeding towards me; it was dark, and I was forced to do some rather evasive driving. Just like in the movies. And just like in the movies, I made all the right moves and was able to zip out of the one way unscathed and undetected by the powers that be! That was way to close! I don't generally head out trying to break the law, but I managed to break a few of them on this night! The rest of the trip home paled in comparison, thank God!

I have a busy day ahead of me but I like it that way. But first, breakfast, and I seem to be on a runaway on the absolute worst day I could pick. Too bad! I'm hungry and I'm eating!

Lots of running around this morning and 2 possessions later make me a very happy boy! And I'm awaiting 1 more possession today. These are problems that I love.

It's time to eat. When isn't it? And we know who gets my business, don't we?

I'm going to really have to be careful the rest of the day. I'm busy, I'm running, and as a result, it's so easy to eat and run, and if I do that, I know I'll screw up. Slow down DD. Relax.

Believe it or not, I haven't shared any of this journey with Malena, other than in very broad strokes. She has told me time and again that she loves me just the way I am. That certainly takes off the pressure but I'm doing this for a lot more than vanity reasons. I have full intentions of being around for a very long time and getting rid of the excess weight is certainly a big part of it.

AFTER 80 DAYS - THE VERDICT

I'm down to 235 pounds (37 pounds in total)! Don't get me wrong; I'm happy but I really, really wanted to hit the 40 pound mark. I could have if I would have just laid off the food for the last couple of days. I just couldn't bring myself to do it just for the numbers. I wanted to, but I didn't, so here I am. Yea me!

So to recap a little: I eat at McD's approximately 90% of the time (the full daily menus are at the back of this book) and yet, I've managed to lose 37 pounds so far in 80 days. I want 40 and I'll get it in the days to come, just wait and see.

I'd come so close! How could I quit now? I needed to lose another 3 pounds. So I made a decision to extend my program a few more days, after all, it might only take a couple more days to hit the numbers I want.

THE FINAL TEN DAYS

Day 81. I am hungry! And as much as I want to get rid of that final 3 pounds, it ain't gonna happen today! I just finished consuming hot cakes and syrup at McD's and it barely made a dent, and that my friends, is not a good thing!

It's time for a road trip which takes me to Falher, Watino, Eaglesham, Grande Prairie, and finally back to Wembley. And did I eat along the way? You bet! Lots, especially in Watino. I'd been invited to lunch and I wasn't about to pass that up. I mean, how could I not eat the baked beans, and the potato salad, and the Kentucky Fried Chicken, as well as the apple pie smothered in whipped cream? I mean, really. A couple of cold beer on the deck and all was well with the world!

I will pay! Guaranteed! But, since I'd already screwed up anyway, I might as well eat a couple of cobs of corn loaded with butter and salt.

That should have been that, but nope. Not today. 2 soft ice cream would complete the binge.

I finally went home, and for the next two hours I sat out on the deck writing to my heart's content. It was pitch black and the coyotes were telling their stories for all the world to hear. It had been a great day. Too bad I had to try and eat myself to death!

Earlier in the day I'd stopped to visit Mom at the Villa in Falher. She'd made a recent decision to move there from the home she and Dad had occupied for the past 10 years. In June of 2012 Dad passed away, and we weren't sure if Mom would move or not. She decided she would stay where she was until she felt it was the right time to move. Fortunately, she was in good health and was able to make the decision when she was good and ready.

But we wondered, how did she really feel about the move? She doesn't always share a lot of information but today was different. She asked me to look at her notebook at what she had written. I read it and I asked her if I could share it on my blog. She reluctantly agreed and I posted it. It is entitled: A CHANGE IS A COMING. Check it out if you're so inclined (www.ddander.com).

Day 82. Forget the weighin this morning. After yesterday's eating disaster the last thing I want to do is step on the scales. Still, I'm not going to beat up on myself too much, after all, I had a good run, and I'll complete the mission in the next few days. Guaranteed!

I think I spoke a little too soon. I did go to McD's for breakfast before heading to church. But then I joined some friends at the Canadian Brewhouse for lunch, and once again, disaster! Get this: I ate a 4 egg omelette, hash browns, and several slices of toast, and then, to add insult to injury, I stopped at McD's for a soft ice cream!

But all was not lost. I had conveniently packed my workout clothes and I decided to put them to good use. Once I get to the trails, I'm away and hopefully I could begin to turn the tide once again.

I made my way home in the early evening, and enjoyed the deck that's becoming my sanctuary where I can write and enjoy the cool breeze that is beckoning the rain to come.

Day 83. I had to head to the hospital this morning for a stress test and to be fitted for a heart monitor, which I have to wear for the next 24 hours. I'm not quite sure why they're insisting on this; I certainly don't have any obvious symptoms. I'm not about to tell anyone as I'm really not in the greatest frame of mind at the moment. I'm irritated, mostly at myself, and I want to have a pity party, and I will, but nobody's invited.

I have to be so careful when I get like this or I'll eat whatever presents itself, and I can guarantee you that it will be straight junk food. And that I do not need. 3 pounds to go . . . 3 pounds to go . . .

I'd rather not see anyone today but in my world, that is an impossibility. And of course, I'll be my usual happy self, as is my norm. I ended up in a great discussion with a couple of people in McD's, and whether I want to admit it or not, I love these discussions.

I headed to CR tonight, which is the perfect place to go given my current state of mind, and shared a whole lot more than I normally do. I guess if one is going to dump junk, that's the place to do it. I headed home shortly thereafter but made one quick pit stop to pick up a bag of cheezies and a pop. Darn!

Day 84. I'm amazed that I haven't gained back a few pounds. I should have, given my eating habits the past few days. Maybe today is the day I begin to turn this all around again.

I have to admit that I'm starting to feel pretty good again. I need to be really careful today so I can get this ship headed in the right direction. I'll still eat at McD's but I'll get back to controlling my portions and I'll definitely cut out the night eating.

The first thing I did was rip off that monitor along with a bunch of hair. Wonderful. And then I went to McD's. I love, love, love breakfast, and I would never deny myself that.

The rest of the day was status quo, and as long as I keep myself busy, I'll do fine. We shall see.

Day 85. I find it hilarious the amount of compliments that I get. "You look great!" If they only knew, and yet I know that's unfair, since I had lost 20 plus pounds and most of these people hadn't seen me in a while. I need to smarten up.

My day was uneventful, and I did manage to make it to the trails for a walk. Slow and steady wins the race, and I am certainly going slow these days!

When I'm in the zone, I do well, and I don't over eat. I'm feeling cautiously optimistic. Maybe I'm back . . .

Day 86. I'm off on another road trip to Falher and area again. I wanted to discuss the Panama situation with Mom but she really isn't open to have that conversation. I know she worries about me, but I'm following my heart, and this is where it's taking me. Right or wrong, it's a decision that I made and I intend on following it through. I hope that one day she will understand that, and realize that I dearly want to talk to her about it. In fact, this is an area of contention with most of my family and it results in a chasm that is proving difficult to traverse. And at some point, the divide will be insurmountable. I pray it will not come to that!

Day 87. Thankfully it was a busy day. That really helps me stay connected and I rarely overeat when I'm engaged as I was today. Boredom does not have a home when I'm busy and thus, I don't overeat.

I was just offered a job near Fox Creek. The call came out of the blue and they would need me to start immediately. Sorry, no can do! I may not be terribly busy at the moment but I still prefer the wonderful world of real estate over the oil patch. I hope I haven't made a huge mistake. There are many who would condemn me for this decision if they knew, but it's my life, and besides, I'm not telling.

In any case, we're moving into our virtual office over the next few days. How does one move into anything that's virtual? I'll have to get back to you on that one. But there is an upside:

expenses go down substantially, and that alone puts me several steps closer to the airport, and I do like to fly!

Day 88. I'm edging ever closer to my goal and I'm starting to get a wee bit excited. I know I can do this, but I also know how easily I can screw it up, so I've got to be extra careful.

I ate at the Golden Arches as usual but I've been pretty good at portion control, and as a result, I'm making progress. The hardest part is the head games which I seem to insist on playing with myself.

I headed to the trails on three separate occasions today. I am determined to win at the losing game, and the trails are the perfect anecdote for me. I win physically, as well as mentally, and when I'm on the trails, I'm definitely not eating.

I'm getting closer and closer. Very soon now. I've lost my IPAD for a couple of days so that's really affecting my writing. My mind speeds along a lot faster than a pen on paper so I just hope I can read my writing when I try to transcribe the past couple of days writing. You may have noticed that the dailies are a little shorter, and now you know why.

Day 89. I am missing Malena big time. God, I wish I could get on that bird and fly away! I guess it'll happen in due course but patience is certainly not my greatest virtue!

Of course, I hit McD's for breakfast and then I headed to church. I really enjoy the services. They help keep me focused on my priorities and on my purpose. And my purpose will require me leading a very long, and healthy life, therefore, I need to lose the excess weight if I expect to be around another hundred years (Ok, maybe not quite that long)!

I've purposely not mentioned my weight the last few days. It's not that I believe in jinx's, but why take any chances. But to ensure success, I'm hitting the trails shortly.

I'm feeling good and I'm feeling strong. I think I've got this, but I'll play this out through Day 90. Then I'll weigh in and accept whatever the results are.

Day 90. The final day. At least, I hope so! Of course, it starts out at McD's as usual. This might turn out to be a tough day as I can already tell that my head is playing games with me. Every time I get close to that final weigh in, the attacks begin. I just pray that I can get through this day without screwing up too much.

The day went excruciatingly slow and the temptations were everywhere. I didn't feel like hitting the trails. I felt like eating everything in sight, but thank God, I didn't.

There wasn't much I could say that was good about this day but it eventually came to an end. Now, if I can just have a good, long sleep followed by a really good weighin, I'll be one happy boy. I guess we'll know in a few hours!

AFTER 90 DAYS - THE VERDICT

Well, the time has come. I adjusted the scales accordingly and took a deep breath, and stepped on. In fact, I stepped on it three separate times just to make sure. The number stayed the same all three times: 232 pounds! Finally!

I began this odyssey at 272 pounds and over 90 days dropped 40 pounds to land at 232 pounds. I'm certainly happy with the results but I know that now the real challenge begins. I weighed 233 pounds when I got my clean bill of health in December of 2011, and was advised by my Doctor that if I continued to make the progress that I was currently making, that he'd likely never have to see me again. What he meant was that I needed to continue dropping the weight, preferably another 30 pounds, keep up the exercise, and definitely never lose my attitude!

I'd like to say that I listened to my doctor, but I didn't. Attitude, yes, but the exercise and the continued weight loss seemed to evade me. And thus, the rest of the story.

I know the critics will take exception to everything I've done up to this point. No surprise there. But, I have made many changes as well. I know my strength was in portion control, and secondly, cutting out the night eating. I fully intended on making some serious changes earlier but I just couldn't do it. As a result, this process is taking a bit longer than I wanted. I have full intentions of eating a lot more fruit and vegetables in the future, and I am fully committed to picking up the exercise quotient substantially. I know I need to do these things, and I will, when I'm ready.

I did what I could do with where I was at at this time in my life. I fully intend on picking up the pace in the days ahead. I'm undergoing a complete lifestyle overhaul, and I'm doing it in a way that is working for me. And I suspect there are a lot of others out there that are just like me.

NOW WHAT?

I decided that I needed to see what would happen if I went back to my "normal" life. I would quit recording my food intake and just go about my daily life as I had before, hoping that I would have learned something about myself over these past 90 days. I knew this was risky as I've been here, done that, on several occasions in the past. 40 pounds were gone and I was 1 pound less than the weight I had dropped to after the surgery. And now I could really go for it (Unfortunately, I didn't)!

Expecting anything different was probably expecting too much from myself, and soon I found myself back in the desert. It was becoming readily apparent why the Israelites took 40 years, not 40 days, to finally make it into the promised land.

At first, it was relatively easy. I ate the breakfast I wanted as I knew the day's business would take care of any excess calories, and I portion controlled anything else I consumed during the day. I also refused to eat anything after dinner, so by 7 pm or so, water or Diet Coke were the only things making it to my mouth. So far, so good.

But, as has happened numerous times before, I began to undo some of the rules I had imposed on myself. Perhaps I could have the popcorn loaded with butter at the movies, after all, it wasn't like I went to the movies every day. And so what if I had a soft ice cream in the evenings once in a while. What's the big deal?

I was regularly being complimented about how good I looked. Thank you very much! But, it went downhill from there. So what if I was up a couple of pounds! I'll just lay off the food for a couple of days and that'll get me back on track. And it did. For a time, but soon it wasn't 2 pounds anymore, now it was 5, and I would promise myself that I would never let it get to 10!

But it did. And then I would bear down and tackle those extra pounds that I had carelessly let find their way back home. I soon found that the 10 pounds I had taken a month to gain back would now take me at least 3 months or more to lose. I persevered and claimed victory again, and then again, and yet again.

After those scares, I had to reevaluate where I was at, and I had to face the fact that even after the 40 pound loss, I still had a long ways to go. After all, when I began this odyssey, my ultimate goal was to settle in around the 200-205 pound mark. Even after the 90 days, I still had 30 more pounds to go, and now I was in danger of making that into 40 or 50 pounds.

Remember, I had open heart surgery and the major recommendation to come out of that was rather simple: continue to lose weight and continue to be as active as you are, and we will probably never see you again! Now here I was again, lost in the desert with absolutely no one to blame but myself.

I know when I began my 40 day program, I had a lot of naysayers telling me how ridiculous I was being. Whatever! But the results spoke for themselves. Of course, it took 2 rounds of 40 days and another 10 days added on to that, but I made it. And that was all that counted.

So I dug in once again, and though I didn't religiously monitor myself over the next few months, I did pay more attention, particularly to my mental state. I spend a lot of time alone, and that can be a dangerous thing. I'm rarely lonely, but it happens, and when it does I need to be careful. I've chosen to run to food as a comforter rather than to drugs, alcohol, women, and so on.

I guess I should be happy about this, and I am for the most part. Still . . .

When the deals are slow to come and when the timetable for my departure seems to grow further away rather than closer, I get anxious and frustrated. Then I console myself, usually with food. And then I hate myself 10 minutes later and I promise myself that tomorrow I'll get back on track.

I know there are millions of others just like me. I know there are billions of dollars spent trying one program after another to get it together, and I know that most of them fail. But still, what choice do we have but to try, and if necessary, try again, and if that fails, try yet again, and again, and again?

I need to constantly remind myself that there are people who care deeply for me, and want me around for a long time, and that I have an obligation to them as well as to my Creator.

I don't understand how I've allowed myself to get to this place yet again when there have been so many "coincidences" happen to me; that to deny them would be to deny God himself! Dramatic! Yes indeed, but also true.

So over the last couple of years or so, I've gained and lost that same 10 pounds at least 4 times. Lately, I find myself slipping even further. Where it was once 10, it's become 15 or more, and I'm finding it harder and harder to rein it in. I thought I'd pick up the exercise quotient a lot more but I haven't been able to maintain it. Mentally I'm exhausted, economically distressed, and the love of my life seems ever farther away. She's not, and she's not going anywhere, but it is taking me forever to get there. And then I eat. And then I feel worse. So I eat some more.

As you can tell, this is an ongoing struggle, though few know about it, as I am one of those guys who everyone thinks has it all together. "DD is always so happy. What an attitude he has! He empowers people around him. He always has time for others." Again, thank you, but I am getting really tired.

But, I do want to live a long, healthy, and active life so I refuse to give up. I just got a call from the cardiologist asking me to come in for a stress test, etc. in, believe it or not, 40 days from now! Seriously, you can't make up this stuff! So, I'm going to use this "coincidence" to kick my butt once again, so when I see the good Doctor I will once again get the "thumbs up" that I don't deserve, but absolutely need.

FINAL NOTE

I had my appointment with the Cardiologist. I had an ECG as well as a stress test. Final BP 140/80. He was happy. So was

I. One note: make sure you keep your weight under control and . . . cut down on the sodium.

It's a never ending story, isn't it?

MY MENU FOR THE LAST 90 DAYS

The first 10 days:

1. 1 Egg McMuffin, 1 cinnamon bun, 1 small fries, 1 peanut butter sandwich, 1 bag of cheezies (100ml), lots of Diet Coke

2. 1 McGriddle, 1 Quarter pounder with cheese, 2 small fries, 1 cheese sandwich, 1 bag of cheezies 100ml), several Diet Coke

3. 1 Sausage and Egg McMuffin, 2 large burgers, 2 slices of ham, 1 fried egg, several slices of cheddar cheese, salad, 1 cheese cake, 1 large serving of Chinese food combo, and several Diet Coke

4. 1 Egg McMuffin, 1 bran muffin, 1 McDouble, 1 small fries, several Diet Coke

5. 1 Egg McMuffin, 1 breakfast burrito, 1 McDouble, 1 small fries, several Diet Coke

6. 1 Egg McMuffin, hash brown, 1 McDouble, 1 small fries, 1 small cone, 1 large dinner at the church, complete with dessert, several Diet Coke

7. 1 Egg McMuffin, 1 hash brown, 2 large plates of stir fry loaded with veggies and chicken, several Diet Coke

8. 1 Egg McMuffin, 1 hash browns, 1 Quarter cheese, 1 medium fries, several Diet Coke

9. 1 Egg McMuffin, 1 hash brown, 1 Quarter pounder with cheese, 1 medium fries, several Diet Coke

10. 1 Egg McMuffin, 1 hash brown, 1 Quarter pounder with cheese, 1 medium fries, lots of Diet Coke

The second 10 days:

1. 1 Egg McMuffin, 1 hash brown, 1 large cheeseburger, fries, and gravy (Falher), lots of Diet Coke

2. 1 Egg McMuffin combo, 1 cheddar and cheese roast beef sandwich and curly fries (Arby's), 1 bran muffin, lots of Diet Coke

3. 1 Bacon, Egg, Cheese McGriddle combo, 2 helpings of lasagna, Caesar salad, apple pie with whipped cream, lots of Diet Coke

4. 1 Bacon, egg, cheese McGriddle combo, 1 Quarter cheese combo, lots of Diet Coke

5. 1 Bacon, Egg, Cheese McGriddle combo, 1 Quarter cheese combo again, lots of Diet Coke

6. The exact same thing as yesterday

7. Once again, the same as above

8. Same again but add 1 banana and lots of water

9. Same once more minus the banana

10. 2 Bacon, Egg, Cheese McGriddles, 1 bran muffin, 2 huge burgers, cheddar, veggies, and desert at The Reach, plus lots of Diet Coke

The third 10 days:

1. 1 McGriddle combo, 1 breakfast burrito, 1 bran muffin, 1 Sweet Chili McWrap, lots of Diet Coke

2. 1 McGriddle combo, 1 Quarter Cheese combo, lots of Diet Coke

3. Same as number two

4. 1 McGriddle combo, 1 Quarter Cheese combo, 2 slices of meat lovers pizza, lots of Diet Coke

5. Bad day. Lots of homemade food all days, lots of Diet Coke.

6. 1 McGriddle combo, 1 Quarter Cheese combo, 1 large buttered popcorn, lots of Diet Coke

7. 1 McGriddle combo, 1 Quarter Cheese combo, lots of Diet Coke

8. Same as yesterday

9. 1 McGriddle combo, 1 Quarter Cheese combo, lots of Diet Coke

10. The exact same thing as yesterday

The fourth 10 days:

1. 1 Bacon, Egg, Cheese McGriddle combo, 2 huge plates of grilled chicken stir fry, lots of Diet Coke

2. 1 Bacon, Egg, Cheese McGriddle, 1 McDouble, small fries, and lots of Diet Coke

3. 1 Bacon, Egg, Cheese McGriddle, 1 breakfast burrito, 1 McDouble, small fries, lots of Diet Coke

4. 1 McGriddle, 1 Sweet Chili McWrap (grilled chicken), 1 McDouble, small fries, and lots of Diet Coke

5. 1 McGriddle, 1 cheeseburger, 1 McDouble, small fries, 1 soft ice cream cone, lots of Diet Coke

6. 1 McGriddle, 1 burrito, 1 Asian salad with grilled chicken , 1 bran muffin, lots of Diet Coke

7. 1 McGriddle, 1 burrito, 1 grilled cheese sandwich, 1 huge burrito loaded, lots of Diet Coke

8. 1 McGriddle, 1 McDouble, small fries, 1 large buttered popcorn, lots of Diet Coke

9. 1 McGriddle, 1 bran muffin, 1 Sweet Chili McWrap, Diet Coke

10. 1 McGriddle, 1 burrito, 1 bran muffin, 1 roast beef with cheese sandwich (Arby's), Diet Coke

The fifth 10 days:

1. 1 McGriddle, 1 McDouble, 1 small fries, 1 bran muffin, Diet Coke

2. 2 McGriddles, turkey dinner, mashed potatoes, gravy, condiments, dessert, and Diet Coke

3. 1 McGriddle, 1 clubhouse, 1 garden salad, 1 McDouble, 1 small fries, 1 large peanut butter sandwich, Diet Coke

4. 1 McGriddle, 1 large Chili and cheese, 1 large soft ice cream, a handful of Cheerios, Diet Coke

5. 1 McGriddle, 1 McDouble, 1 small fries, roasted chicken, carrots, peas, rice, dessert, cheezies, Diet Coke

6. 2 eggs, toast, bacon, 2 bagels, peanut butter and jam, 1 huge cheeseburger, fries, and gravy, soup, Diet Coke

7. 1 McGriddle, 1 Egg McMuffin, 1 bran muffin, 1 large buttered popcorn, Diet Coke

8. 1 McGriddle, 1 salmon sandwich, cheddar, ice tea, pickles, Diet Coke

9. 1 McGriddle, 1 burrito, 2 bananas, 1 McDouble, 1 small fries, Diet Coke, and lots of water

10. 1 McGriddle, 1 burrito, 1 McDouble, 1 small fries, 1 tablespoon of peanut butter, Diet Coke

The sixth 10 days:

1. 2 McGriddles, 1 McDouble, 1 small fries, 1 soft ice cream, 1 large peanut butter sandwich, 1 handful of cashews, 1 handful of almonds, Diet Coke

2. 2 McGriddles, 1 Sweet Chili McWrap with grilled chicken, 1 small fries, Diet Coke

3. 1 McGriddle, 1 Egg McMuffin, 1 grilled chicken breast at home, mixed veggies, a handful of mixed nuts, Diet Coke

4. 1 McGriddle, 1 Egg McMuffin, 1 soft ice cream, 1 grilled chicken breast, mixed veggies, Diet Coke

5. 2 McGriddles, 1 lemon salmon fillet with veggies and salad, 1 soft ice cream, 2 beer, Diet Coke

6. 2 Egg McMuffins, 1 McDouble, 1 small fries, Diet Coke

7. 1 Egg McMuffin with an extra egg, 1 fruit parfait, 1 fruit and nut protein bar, lots of water, 1 Sweet Chili McWrap with grilled chicken, 1 skinless chicken breast, Diet Coke

8. 1 Bacon and Egg McMuffin with an extra egg, 1 Sweet Chili McWrap, 1 McDouble, 1 small fries, 1 tablespoon of peanut butter, Diet Coke

9. 1 Egg McMuffin with an extra egg, 1 burrito, 1 grilled chicken wrap, 1 medium buttered popcorn, 1 tablespoon of peanut butter, Diet Coke

10. 1 Egg McMuffin with an extra egg, 1 McDouble, 1 small fries, 1 soft ice cream, 1 chicken breast, veggies, Diet Coke

The seventh 10 days:

1. 1 Bacon and Egg McMuffin, 1 grapefruit, 1 Double cheeseburger, 1 small fries, 1 large cheeseburger and fries at Tony Roma's, 1 banana, 1 protein bar, Diet Coke

2. 1 Egg McMuffin with an extra egg, 1 banana, 3 burgers and potato salad, 1 chocolate bar, 1 bran muffin, Diet Coke

3. 1 McGriddle, 1 Asian salad with grilled chicken, 1 McDouble, 1 small fries, Diet Coke

4. 1 McGriddle, 3 pieces of fish and chips at Joeys, 2 huge dishes of stir fry with grilled chicken, Diet Coke

5. 1 Egg McMuffin with an extra egg, 1 turkey wrap, 1 grilled chicken snack wrap, 1 small soft ice cream, Diet Coke

6. 1 Egg McMuffin with an extra egg, 1 grilled chicken snack wrap, a plate of roast beef and Kraft dinner, 1 grapefruit, lots of water today

7. 1 Egg McMuffin with an extra egg, 1 burrito, 1 Asian salad with grilled chicken, 1 McDouble, 1 small fries, Diet Coke

8. 1 Egg McMuffin with an extra egg, 1 burrito, 1 Quarter cheese combo, 1 soft ice cream, Diet Coke

9. 1 Egg McMuffin with an extra egg, 2 protein bars, Diet Coke

10. 1 Egg McMuffin with an extra egg, 2 grilled chicken snack wraps, Diet Coke

The eighth 10 days:

1. 1 Egg McMuffin with an extra egg, 1 burrito, 2 snack wraps with grilled chicken, Diet Coke

2. 1 Egg McMuffin with an extra egg, 1 burrito, 1 bowl of chicken noodle soup, 3/4 head of raw cabbage, a few chunks of kohlrabi, Diet Coke

3. 1 Egg McMuffin with an extra egg, 1 burrito, 1 plate of chicken souvlaki at Tito's, Diet Coke

4. 1 Egg McMuffin with an extra egg, 1 burrito, a huge dinner consisting of steak, potatoes, peppers, mushrooms, salad, Saskatoon pie and ice cream, a glass of wine, Diet Coke

5. 1 Egg McMuffin with an extra egg, 1 burrito, 1 smoothie, 1 loaded hotdog, 1 slice pepperoni pizza, 2 cones, 1 bran muffin, 1 snack wrap, 1 small bag of cheezies, Diet Coke

6. 1 Egg McMuffin with an extra egg, 2 grilled chicken snack wraps, Diet Coke

7. 2 Egg McMuffins with extra eggs, 2 snack wraps with grilled chicken, Diet Coke

8. 2 Egg McMuffins and extra eggs, 1 Sweet Chili McWrap with grilled chicken, Diet Coke

9. 1 Egg McMuffin with an extra egg, 1 burrito, 1 soft ice cream, 1 grilled chicken snack wrap, Diet Coke

10. 2 Egg McMuffins with extra eggs, 1 McDouble, 1 small fries, Diet Coke

The ninth 10 days:

1. 1 hot cakes and syrup, baked beans, potato salad, KFC chicken (4 pieces), salad, apple pie and whipped cream, 2 cobs of buttered corn, 1 beer, 2 soft ice cream, Diet Coke

2. 1 four egg omelette, hash browns, toast, 1 grilled chicken snack wrap, 1 soft ice cream, Diet Coke

3. 1 Egg McMuffin with an extra egg, 1 cheeseburger and fries, 1 soft ice cream, 1 bran muffin, 1 large bag of cheezies, Diet Coke

4. 1 Egg McMuffin with an extra egg, 1 burrito, 2 McDoubles and fries, 1 small bag of cheezies, Diet Coke

5. 1 Egg McMuffin with an extra egg, 1 burrito, 1 grilled chicken snack wrap, Diet Coke

6. 2 Egg McMuffins with extra eggs, 1 burrito, 1 soft ice cream, 1 grilled chicken snack wrap, 1 McDouble with fries, 1 large bag of cheezies, 1 chocolate bar, Diet Coke

7. 1 Egg McMuffin with an extra egg, 1 burrito, 1 McDouble with fries, 1 soft ice cream, Diet Coke

8. 1 Egg McMuffin with an extra egg, 1 burrito, 1 McDouble and small fries, 1 small cone, Diet Coke

9. 1 Egg McMuffin with an extra egg, 1 burrito, boiled cabbage, roast beef, pea soup, 1 beer, salad, some boiled potatoes, Diet Coke

10. 1 Egg McMuffin with an extra egg, 1 grilled chicken snack wrap, 1 McDouble, Diet Coke

And there you have it! This may drive others insane, but this is what I ate and drank over the last 90 days; in addition, I drank large quantities of water daily. I have to admit, I still enjoy this type of food immensely!

ABOUT THE AUTHOR

DD ANDER never did fit in very well in the prairie town he grew up in. While his classmates were settling down to careers and raising families, he was dreaming of mountain peaks and tall ships. And though he would attempt to follow these dreams, he would always end up back home on the prairies.

For a good part of his life he stayed the course, but eventually, he took his leave. He travelled extensively, and his experiences would soon catch up with his passion for a different life.

It would take him to places he should not have trod, and into experiences he should not have had. Stories would be told, by him, that he would deem fiction, but those who knew him, knew not where the fiction ended and the truth began. And they dared not ask.

He began to blog regularly during this time. Hundreds of blogs would follow, and to those who knew him well, it became obvious that the greater story lie between the lines. The public story was there for all the world to see, the other, for certain eyes only.

Although he lives in another part of the world today, he is always close by in one form or another. Whether through his blogs, photos, novels (both fiction and non fiction), or one on one conversations, he is never very far away.

My website is:

www.ddander.com

ISBN number: 978-0-9953193-2-5

www.ingramcontent.com/pod-product-compliance
Lightning Source LLC
Chambersburg PA
CBHW071125280326
41935CB00010B/1114